High Frequency Ventilation

Editors

Lyle H. Hamilton, Ph.D.
Professor
Department of Physiology
Medical College of Wisconsin
and Principal Scientist
Department of Research Service
Zablocki VA Medical Center
Milwaukee, Wisconsin

Josef Neu, M.D.
Associate Professor
Department of Pediatrics
University of Florida
Gainesville, Florida

Jerry M. Calkins, M.D., Ph.D.
Associate Professor
Vice Chairman
Department of Anesthesiology
University of North Carolina
School of Medicine
Chapel Hill, North Carolina

CRC Press, Inc.
Boca Raton, Florida

Library of Congress Cataloging-in-Publication Data
Main entry under title:

High frequency ventilation.

Includes bibliographies and index.
1. Artificial respiration. 2. Ventilation.
3. Respiratory therapy. I. Hamilton, Lyle H.,
1924— . II. Neu, Josef. III. Calkins, Jerry M.
[DNLM: 1. Respiration, Artificial, WF 145 H6379]
RC87.9.H54 1986 615.8'36 85-31355
ISBN-0-8493-6739-5

Direct all inquiries to CRC Press, Inc., 2000 Corporate Blvd., N.W., Boca Raton, Florida, 33431.

International Standard Book Number 0-8493-6739-5

Library of Congress Card Number 85-31355
Printed in the United States

PREFACE

The introduction of mechanical ventilation to medicine has saved many lives. Improvements in ventilator design have made them even more effective in recent decades. More recently, the introduction of mechanical ventilation at frequencies much greater than those generated during spontaneous breathing have been demonstrated to offer good CO_2-elimination, adequate O_2-delivery, and improved central hemodynamics in patients with disease processes. The interest and enthusiasm which that observation stimulated is apparent from the numerous publications in the area within the past few years. Scientists and physicians have been investigating the mechanism of how ventilation can be accomplished with tidal volumes less than anatomic dead space, as well as searching for disease entities where the application of this new technique would be most beneficial.

This book was assembled in an effort to summarize some of the information which has been gained in the area of high frequency ventilation (HFV) from both a basic science and an applied science point of view. We have attempted to include potential applications to neonates and children, as well as to adults, and to address a few selected topics, such as new types of ventilators, effects of HFV on gas exchange in the lung, and on alterations in the regulation of breathing. We think the topics are timely and we hope the book serves its readers well.

The Editors would like to thank the contributing authors and the publishers, for their patience and understanding during this exercise.

Lyle H. Hamilton
Jerry M. Calkins
Josef Neu

THE EDITORS

Lyle H. Hamilton, Ph.D. is Professor of Physiology in the Medical College of Wisconsin and Principal Research Scientist for the Zablocki VA Medical Center, both in Milwaukee, Wisconsin.

He obtained an A.B. degree in Biology from Willamette University, Salem Oregon, and M.S. and Ph.D. degrees in Physiology from the State University of Iowa. He was on the faculty in the Department of Physiology at the University of Saskatchewan before coming to Milwaukee in 1957. Dr. Hamilton's research interests are in respiratory physiology and instrumentation. In these and associated areas, he has published over 100 papers and over 60 abstracts. He is co-author of a textbook on Respiratory Physiology, written with N.B. Slonim, M. D., has been on research review-boards, contributed to medical education in the Caribbean for over 15 years, and participated in graduate student and post-doctoral training for 30 years.

Dr. Hamilton is a member of several professional organizations, including the American Physiological Society, Canadian Physiological Society, American College of Sports Medicine, and Biomedical Engineering Society.

Jerry M. Calkins received his B.S. and M.S. degrees in chemical engineering from the University of Wyoming. After a tour of duty with the U.S. Army at the Harry Diamond Laboratories where he served as the Director of the Biomedical Engineering Section, he obtained his Ph.D. in chemical engineering from the University of Maryland. He subsequently joined the engineering faculty at Arizona State University. Because of his interest in technology in medicine, he chose to study medicine and received his M.D. from the University of Arizona. After completing his residency in anesthesiology at the University of Arizona, he accepted a faculty position in the Department of Anesthesiology with a joint appointment to the Clinical Engineering Program of the College of Engineering. Dr. Calkins is currently an Associate Professor and the Vice Chairman of the Department of Anesthesiology at the University of North Carolina School of Medicine.

Dr. Calkins is author of numerous scientific publications and book chapters. His principal areas of interest involve both the biomedical engineering and medical disciplines, with studies in development of life-support systems and implementation of technology for anesthesia delivery systems and monitoring. Dr. Calkins is a member of several medical and engineering professional societies, and has been the recipient of many awards and honors, including a National Science Foundation Fellowship, a National Institutes of Health Special Fellowship, and the Upjohn Achievement Award for Outstanding Educator.

Josef Neu, M.D. is Associate Professor of Pediatrics at the University of Florida in Gainesville, Florida. Dr. Neu obtained his M.D. degree at the University of Wisconsin, completed his pediatric residency at Johns Hopkins University Medical Center in 1978, and completed his fellowship in neonatology at Stanford University Medical Center in 1980. He also served on the faculty at the Medical College of Wisconsin for 3½ years before joining the faculty of the University of Florida. Dr. Neu is the Associate Division Chief of the Division of Neonatology and the Co-Director of the Pediatric Intensive Care Unit at the University of Florida Shands Hospital. He is a member of the Society of Critical Care Medicine and the American Academy of Pediatrics. He has authored/coauthored approximately 40 articles, abstracts, and chapters related to pediatrics, several of them in the area of neonatal ventilation.

CONTRIBUTORS

Desmond J. Bohn, M.B., B.Ch., F.R.C.P.(C)
Assistant Director
Intensive Care Unit
Hospital for Sick Children
and
Assistant Professor of Anesthesia
University of Toronto
Toronto, Ontario, Canada

A. Charles Bryan, M.B., B.S., Ph.D., F.R.C.P.(C)
Professor of Anesthesia and Pediatrics
Department of Respiratory Physiology
Hospital for Sick Children
Toronto, Ontario, Canada

Richard L. Bucciarelli, M.D.
Associate Professor
Chief, Division of Neonatology
Department of Pediatrics
University of Florida
Gainesville, Florida

Jerry M. Calkins, M.D., Ph.D.
Associate Professor and Vice Chairman
Department of Anethesiology
University of Arizona Medical Center
Tucson, Arizona

Graziano C. Carlon, M.D.
Clinical Chief
Department of Critical Care
Memorial Sloan-Kettering Cancer Center
New York, New York

H. K. Chang, Ph.D.
Professor
Department of Biomedical Engineering
and
Department of Physiology and Biophysics
University of Southern California
Los Angeles, California

Jacqueline J. Coalson, Ph.D.
Professor
Department of Pathology
University of Texas Health Sciences Center
San Antonio, Texas

Arthur H. Combs, M.D.
Senior Research Fellow
Department of Critical Care
Memorial Sloan-Kettering Cancer Center
New York, New York
and presently
Director of Critical Care
Providence Hospital
Washington, D.C.

Robert A. DeLemosh, M.D.
Chairman
Department of Physiology and Medicine
Southwest Foundation for Biomedical Research
San Antonio, Texas

Sandra J. England, Ph.D.
Assistant Professor
Department of Pediatrics
Hospital for Sick Children
Toronto, Ontario, Canada

Erik A. Hagen, M.D.
Research Fellow
Cardiovascular Research Institute
and
Department of Anesthesia
University of California at San Francisco
San Francisco, California

Lyle H. Hamilton, Ph.D.
Professor
Department of Physiology
Medical College of Wisconsin
and
Principal Scientist
Research Service
Zablocki Veterans Administration
Medical Center
Milwaukee, Wisconsin

Wayne Mitzner, Ph.D.
Professor
Division of Environmental Physiology
The Johns Hopkins University
Baltimore, Maryland

Josef Neu, M.D.
Associate Professor of Pediatrics
and Associate Division Chief
Division of Neonatology
University of Florida College of
Medicine
Gainesville, Florida

Donald M. Null, Jr., M.D.
Chief of Neonatology
Department of Pediatrics
Wilford Hall US Air Force Medical
Center
Lackland Air Force Base
San Antonio, Texas

Stuart F. Quan, M.D.
Associate Professor of Internal
Medicine
Division of Respiratory Sciences
University of Arizona College of
Medicine
Tucson, Arizona

Masa Tamura, M.D.
Fellow
Intensive Care Unit
The Hospital for Sick Children
Toronto, Ontario, Canada

Peter D. Wagner, M.D.
Professor of Medicine
Department of Medicine
University of California, San Diego
La Jolla, California

Charles K. Waterson, M.S.E.E.
Biomedical Research Engineer
Department of Anesthesiology
School of Medicine
University of North Carolina
Chapel Hill, North Carolina

TABLE OF CONTENTS

Chapter 1

HISTORICAL DEVELOPMENT OF HIGH FREQUENCY VENTILATION

Lyle H. Hamilton

High frequency ventilation (HFV) is a generic term defining very diverse modalities of assisted ventilation having little in common except elevated frequency and reduced tidal volume. For this reason, even a definition of the term is difficult. Some authors have considered anything over 60 breaths/min as HFV in adults. This is near the normal breathing frequency for neonates. Some workers have proposed that the pattern should achieve a frequency equal to or greater than four times the normal resting rate for that subject. This would require a frequency of 240 or more for it to be classified as HFV in neonates, but many investigators successfully employ a frequency of 150/min in such patients. Mitzner has argued that the common denominator is not high frequency, but rather, reduced tidal volume (see Chapter 2). Whatever the criteria or definition, workers recognize HFV as assisted ventilation with an accelerated frequency and a tidal volume less than that which one would intuitively expect could support adequate gas exchange.

There are four distinct methods of applying HFV, three of which are used in clinical medicine and the fourth, as yet, still an experimental technique.

High frequency positive pressure ventilation (HFPPV) was the first kind of HFV to be described and carefully studied. It uses a ventilator with a small tidal volume (usually 3 to 4 mℓ/kg body weight) and a frequency of 60 to 100 c/min. This requires a system with a small internal dead space in order to keep the internal compliance of the ventilator low and minimize compression of the gases within the ventilator. Peak inspiratory airway pressure is low because tidal volume is small, so lung expansion is not great.

High frequency oscillatory ventilation (HFOV) is based on a cycle frequency of 900 to 3600 c/min (15 to 60 c/s, or Hz). The source of the oscillatory flow may be a piston pump or a large oscillating diaphragm (like a loudspeaker). Both of these devices produce an alternating positive and negative pressure at their output. It results in an oscillatory pattern with no net bulk flow. A bias flow at the oscillator (across the connector to the endotracheal tube) is used to provide fresh gas for ventilation. A different device, which is not really an oscillator but is generally used in the same frequency range, is a rotating valve which interrupts a constant flow. It provides a positive inflation and a passive (rather than negative) deflation phase. Tidal volume is extremely low in all forms of HFOV, ranging from 1 to 3 mℓ/kg body weight under normal circumstances. There is little pressure pulsation, but mean airway pressure must be maintained at a level similar to that used with other ventilators.

High frequency jet ventilation (HFJV) depends on the principle of a jet injector, in which air is entrained by a high velocity pulse of air or oxygen through a narrow cannula in the airway or endotracheal tube. The frequency is usually intermediate between those used in HFPPV and HFOV, as are tidal volume and airway pressure pulses.

The fourth method of applying HFV is high frequency chest wall oscillation (HFCWO), in which a rigid harness, or shell, surrounds the chest and is inflated at frequencies ranging from 3 to 10 Hz. The baseline inflation pressure and cycle volume are adjusted to provide an appropriate tidal volume for the elevated frequency used. A variant of that method is called high frequency body surface oscillation (HFBSO). When it is used, the body is enclosed in an air-tight tank and a reciprocating pump oscillates the pressure about a mean — which may be negative if desired.

At one time, HFV techniques were differentiated on the basis of frequency. That is, HFPPV was HFV in the range of 60 to 100 breaths/min, HFJV was HFV in the 1.5 to 4 c/s (Hz) range and HFOV was HFV at greater than 10 Hz. However, confusion resulted because the ranges sometimes overlapped, and the fundamental characteristics were affected by the devices used, e.g., the rotary interrupter eliminated negative pressure "oscillations" which are characteristic of other kinds of HFOV. Thus, the field has moved away from categories named on the basis of the frequency range, but a universally acceptable classification system has not yet been developed. Dr. Alison Froese has proposed a classification based on whether the expiratory phase of the cycle is active or passive.[1] Those devices with an "active" expiration employ a system which aids expiration, e.g., a piston pump, a bellows or a diaphragm. The HFV-passive ventilators use active inspiration which is interrupted and permits expiration to be passive. They include jet ventilators, the rotating valve, and conventional ventilators used for HFPPV. Ventilators which are ordinarily "passive" can be converted to active expiration by applying a negative pressure to the expiratory line. This approach has been used in laboratory studies with an interruptor (rotating valve) or a jet ventilator by investigators in Baltimore.[103] Its action does not match the active suction provided by a piston pump, but it can definitely assist expiration during the application of higher frequency HFV.

The classification proposed by Froese is attractive on the basis that it has a functional/physiologic basis, but it has not yet been widely accepted, and will require that the frequency be specified in order to define ventilatory assistance in sufficiently exact terms. Perhaps it will always be necessary to also specify the kind of mechanical system employed; to describe the wave-form and to provide information as to whether or not positive end-expiratory pressure was applied, an accepted humidification system was used, and appropriate safety precautions (particularly against accidental over-pressure) were in place.

The history of HFV is not old, but it is surrounded by some lessons to be learned about observations and alertness. The first interesting observation is that it was seen and missed by several astute investigators. The second is that those who did recognize its potential for ventilating patients were using it for something else at the time. In 1915, Henderson et al.[2] indicated that gas exchange could proceed with tidal volumes smaller than dead space volume, and demonstrated that air moved with a parabolic velocity profile through a tube, so fresh air could reach the other end with a smaller flushing volume than the anatomical dead space. This observation was used many years later by Briscoe et al.[3] to explain their observation that a surprisingly small tidal volume (as low as 60 mℓ) could support gas exchange if the breathing frequency was high enough. The information was available in their data to permit these astute investigators to describe high frequency ventilation, but they left for others the excitement of uncovering the principles, defining them by experimental physiology and characterizing them through clinical medicine. Many other physiologists who worked with panting animals or who measured dead space in a variety of experiments must also, have developed data to suggest that gas exchange can occur when the tidal volume is less than dead space if breathing frequency is high enough. In 1962 our own laboratory demonstrated in a totally unrelated study that vertical whole-body vibration at frequencies up to 7 Hz resulted in hyperventilation in healthy volunteers.[4] The response was considered to be mediated directly by mass momentum and indirectly through reflexes of the pulmonary stretch receptors; and the possibility of an effect on airway mixing was not even entertained.

A group of investigators headed by Ulf Sjostrand needed a technique for ventilating animals without producing an effect on the circulatory system. The "Traube-Hering" waves are variations in blood pressure synchronous with breathing, which exerted a disturbing effect on experimental studies of the carotid sinus reflex. Between 1967 and 1971 Sjostrand's team developed HFPPV and demonstrated its ability to provide adequate ventilation without compromising the systemic circulation (or the circulatory reflexes). They were impressed by the ability of this technique to ventilate the animals while avoiding cardiovascular effects, so they began to examine the system for its ventilatory characteristics. Thus began a series of studies which has brought HFPPV to the attention of respiratory physiologists and clinicians world-wide. Their story is chronicled in many articles, and is well represented in reviews by Dr. Sjostrand.[5-7]

Lunkenheimer et al.,[9] in 1972, studied the effect of pericardial pressure oscillations on cardiac performance in a protocol which required apnea during periods of transtracheal pressure oscillations applied to the pericardium. They relied on "diffusion respiration", first described by Draper and Whitehead[8] for oxygenation during the apneic period, and observed that when oscillations of 10 to 20 mℓ volume at a frequency of 23 to 40 Hz were applied transtracheally during those periods, oxygenation was better than when oscillations were not present. Oxygenation was not sensitive to the frequency employed, but clearance of CO_2 was dependent on both frequency and amplitude.[9,10] The authors proposed that the oscillations could provide prolonged "rested" ventilation without thoracic excursions, and their observations led directly to the studies which spawned HFOV. Much credit for the development of HFOV should go to the Toronto group headed by A. C. Bryan. Bohn et al.[11] reported work with animals, which lead to the application of HFOV to humans by Butler et al.,[12] with the demonstration that oscillations of 80 mℓ volume at the mouth, at a cycle frequency of 15 Hz, could be used to maintain arterial P_{O_2} and P_{CO_2}.

Ventilatory assistance by the introduction of a cyclic jet of oxygen at physiological frequencies through a small cannula was introduced by Sanders in 1967[13] to assist bronchoscopy. It was limited to use with bronchoscopy for 10 years, until Klain and Smith[14] combined that delivery method with a transtracheal technique of introducing the cannula, and with the use of a cycle frequency up to 200/min (patterned after the Swedish school). They believed it was a particularly useful technique in CPR.[15] They demonstrated in dogs that gas exchange was adequate, peak inspiratory pressure was low and ventilator-induced circulatory impairment was abolished. Because of their innovative work, questions were raised about the classical beliefs concerning V_D/V_T. Smith and Klain[16] extended the range to 600/min (10 Hz) in dogs, but reported adverse circulatory effects above 400/min. On the basis of that report, most studies of HFJV have been limited to less than 400 c/min. Klain and co-workers and Carlon et al. working together and independently, soon applied HFJV to clinical cases.[15,18-26] Of course, many other laboratories have also helped in the clinical and scientific development of this unique system for providing pulses to assist or control ventilation.

Much attention has been paid to the mechanics of the delivery systems, i.e., ventilators and endotracheal tubes,[24,27-35] and to the mechanism of its action.[36-40] Some of that has resulted from the fact that many laboratories have worked with HFJV, and some is also because the jet injector is not well understood for this application, and deserves more clarification.

Studies of its clinical application and effectiveness have been widespread and prolific for a technique which is so new. HFJV has been demonstrated to be an effective method for ventilating the lungs when there are serious "leaks" in the airway system, such as bronchopleural fistulae[19,35,41-43] or during surgery involving the airways, at which time major bronchi may be totally open.[44-47] Use of percutaneous transtracheal HFJV in CPR was pioneered by Klain and co-workers, and has been studied by others.[28,48] Whether it will move beyond the field of emergency medicine is still conjectural.

Work remains to be done in the area of selecting the most responsive patients, defining optimum operating conditions, developing the most reliable delivery systems and providing maximum safety during the application of jet ventilation.

Chang has been a leader in the development of HFCWO and HFBSO, and has demonstrated their effectiveness in laboratory animals as small as the rat[49] and as large as the dog.[50] Ward et al.[51] have demonstrated the ability of the technique to support gas exchange in the rabbit. It is generally recognized that this method is not likely to be a clinically useful technique for the application of HFV, but it may provide information about mucociliary clearance unattainable with other techniques, or about gas-mixing in the airways when they are not subjected to perturbation by a ventilatory system. Chang and Harf[52] have recently demonstrated that mucociliary clearance may be more effective with HFCWO than with HFOV, and Chang, (Chapter 5) has suggested that the technique may serve as an effective pulsatile assistant to the heart if it is properly synchronized.

HFV has been used with neonates ever since its development. The first study describing the application of HFOV to humans included a 3-day-old infant as a subject.[12] An early reference to the use of HFV for neonates was published as an abstrated by Frantz et al.[53]

They successfully used an Emerson ball-valve interruptor for periods of 1 hr at frequencies up to 30 Hz, with an optimum of 15 to 20 Hz, in premature infants with severe respiratory failure. Their studies were expanded to include its use in the respiratory distress syndrome (RDS) and in pulmonary interstitial emphysema.[54] The application of HFV to RDS has been addressed successfully by several investigators using HFPPV,[55] HFOV,[54,56-58] HFJV,[59-61] or HFJV combined with intermittent mandatory ventilation (IMV).[62] In addition, it has been used successfully with diaphragmatic hernia,[61-63] bronchopleural fistulae,[60] and pulmonary interstitial emphysema.[60,64] A workshop devoted to a study of HFV for immature infants[56] concluded that if HFV is used in neonatology it should probably be used only for investigative work until more questions about the technique and its physiological consequences have been answered. DeLemos from San Antonio has proposed the same restriction,[64] and has suggested that since the success rate with conventional treatment of RDS is high, HFV should probably currently be limited to animal studies on RDS, and then only in institutions having previous experience with animal research in this area. In support of that position, de Lemos is conducting carefully controlled studies toward baboon neonates with induced lung disease. Similar work on premature primates has been reported by Truog et al.[65] Most investigators believe that an exception exists, whereby it is justified to use HFOV for the treatment of pulmonary interstitial emphysema in infants because other approaches are not only unsuccessful, but may aggravate the problem. The justification for using HFJV in neonates has been questioned by some investigators. No advantages of HFJV over HFOV or HFPPV has been demonstrated for ventilatory assistance in neonates, and some suggestions have been made[60,61,64] that damage to the fragile airways of the newborn resulted from either a high velocity of air flow at the outlet of the endotracheal tube, from the temperature of the jet stream (heated by friction or cooled by the adiabatic effect of the expanding gas) or from the inability to fully humidify the gases delivered to the airways.

At least early in the development of HFV it was proposed that one of its major advantages over conventional ventilatory assistance was a reduced airway pressure, with a reduced danger of barotrauma.[7,38] The consequent reduction of intracranial pressure (ICP) and the avoidance of large swings in ICP would be of great benefit in avoiding intracranial hemorrhage in neonates with RDS who are, by necessity, subjected to high inspiratory pressures during ventilatory assistance. Although the peak inspiratory pressure (PIP) may be reduced with all forms of HFV, recent evidence suggests that mean airway pressure (MAP) must be maintained at almost the identical level as with conventional ventilatory assistance to achieve adequate oxygenation,[17,57,66,67] though some investigators report adequate O_2-exchange with lower MAP during HFJV.[59] Operating conditions can modify those airway pressures due to changes in the patient, as demonstrated by Calkins et al.,[68] Carlon et al.,[69] and by Hamilton et al.,[40] with an engineering model. The requirement for maintaining mean P_{aw} at the same level is probably related to the requirement of maintaining lung volume equal to at least FRC, from which gas exchange takes place.

Fourty-four percent of the premature infants who required intensive care were demonstrated by Ahmann et al.[70] to have subependymal or intraventricular hemorrhage (IVH). Dykes et al.[71] also reported significant correlations between IVH and peak inflation pressures above 25 cm H_2O, and between IVH and mechanical ventilation if the patient had RDS. It has been demonstrated that ventilator-induced ICP waveforms were abolished by HFOV[72] and that ICP remained low during a 2-hr session with HFOV. Toutant et al.[73] demonstrated that cerebral blood flow was unaffected by HFV. Carlo et al.[59] reported a decrease in PIP and MAP in RDS patients ventilated with HFJV. Grasberger et al.,[74] on the other hand, demonstrated that mean ICP was the same between HFOV (Emerson rotary valve) and conventional ventilation. Although peak ICP was less with HFOV in a canine head-injury model, it offered no advantages in survival nor in the avoidance of complications associated with elevated ventilatory pressures. The model was not developed to study neonates, however, and it was for the study of ICP rather than RDS. The theoretical advantages of HFV still exist, and results are apparently better with HFOV than with conventional ventilation for RDS, according to most reports in which comparisons were made, so at least part of its superiority may be related to its effect of minimizing peak intracranial pressure.

Theories about how gas exchange can be accommodated with $V_D/V_T > 1.0$ have emanated from many sources. Laboratories from engineering schools and clinics from hospitals have proposed simple and/or elegant theories to reassure us about the violation of concepts we have lived with comfortably for nearly 100 years. Even so, the field has not yet completely defined its terms, and it is not yet able to offer a unified explanation of how HFV "works". Part of the problem is related to inadequate measurement techniques — most pneumotachometers are not fast enough to respond accurately to the high frequencies employed; techniques for measuring pressures within the airways are usually inadequate or they can change the pressure; high air velocities prevent the use of conventional scanning techniques; there is not yet agreement about all the measurements which should be made, or the importance of making them simultaneously. In spite of that, great advances in monitoring, and in experimental data collecting, have been made in a short period of time, and advancements in techniques and instrumentation have contributed greatly to the ability of engineering scientists to propose explanations and to check them out with data.

Ventilation in the physiologic range combines convection and diffusion. Convection (bulk flow) occurs in the larger airways where there is a finite net movement of air. When air is carried to small airways, the velocity of flow is reduced to an insignificant level because of the large cross-sectional area of the multitudinous peripheral airways. From that point to the alveoli, diffusion is responsible for the net movement of any gas species, e.g., CO_2 moves from the region of higher concentration in the alveoli to lower concentration in the small bronchioles, due solely to the CO_2-pressure difference. Simultaneously, O_2 moves from the bronchioles to the alveoli only by diffusion down a concentration gradient.

Convection in the largest airways is probably in the form of turbulent flow, with a flat velocity profile and a moving front which mixes by chaotic eddy currents. Convective flow in smaller (more numerous) airways is considered to be laminar, with a parabolic velocity profile. This type of flow sets up conditions for enhanced, or augmented, gas mixing in the airways. Cardiogenic mixing[75] contributes to airway mixing by the mechanical effect of the heart beat oscillating and vibrating the airways. The principle is widely accepted, though Drechsler and Ultman[76] have shown that the degree of mixing induced by cardiogenic oscillation is independent of the heart rate. Slutsky[77] has predicted that cardiac oscillations can enhance gas mixing 10-fold in the airway of the dog. Slutsky et al.[78] included laminar flow in the peripheral lung units as a condition for airway mixing. They presented evidence that $\dot{V}_{CO_2}$ was proportional to the product of frequency and tidal volume ($f \times V_T$) through a frequency range of 4 to 30 Hz and a tidal volume range equal to 20 to 85% of V_D. They explained their observations on the basis of coupled effects of molecular diffusion and convection (augmented gas transport). In small airways with laminar flow, in addition to axial mixing along the length of the airway, the phenomenon of Taylor dispersion promotes radial mixing in adjacent annular rings which have a concentration gradient due to streamline flow. It is the radial diffusion which is defined as enhanced mixing by Taylor dispersion, and which leads to an apparent bidirectionality for flow. The component with higher alveolar concentration appears to move toward the mouth along the edges of the airway while the component with higher mouth concentration provides the impression of moving toward the alveoli through the center of the stream. Both movements can be explained on the basis of radial diffusion. At the end of an inspiration the tongue of the pulse extends down the airway. It contains relatively higher P_{O_2}, so O_2 diffuses outward to the wall and CO_2 (in higher concentrations toward the alveoli) diffuses in to the center. During the expiratory phase of the cycle, the CO_2-rich air is carried toward the mouth. During that phase the O_2 diffuses into the tongue of the pulse and CO_2 diffuses out. This procedure is repeated many times per second, so each pulse has to account for net flow through only a very short distance for the total mixing to be augmented and for a concentration gradient to be established in the airways.

Fredberg[79] used a semi-empirical analysis to show that augmented diffusion in the central airways was in the form of turbulent mixing, and that when it was combined with molecular diffusion in the peripheral airways, it could account for most gas transport observed during small tidal volumes. In support of Fredberg's concept, Knopp et al.[80] concluded that gas mixing during HFV is not significantly limited by diffusion, so Taylor dispersion could not be a major determinant of airway mixing. On the other hand, Robertson et al.[81] demonstrated an effect of gas density on inert gas elimination, which would not have been predicted from Fredberg's proposal. Khoo et al.,[82] derived a model for transport which also incorporated effective diffusivity and asymmetrical branching networks. In that model, V_T has an additional, independent effect on mixing, in addition to that related to the product of $f \times V_T$. It has been demonstrated by several other investigators[83-85] that HFOV is affected more by tidal volume than by frequency, so a model based only on Taylor dispersion is inadequate to explain gas mixing in the airways during HFV. Solway et al.[86] and Knopp et al.[80] found no effect of changing viscosity and density on gas transport, suggesting that molecular diffusion was also not a major mechanism. On the other hand, Goldman and McDonald[87] and Brusasco et al.[88] did observe an effect of gas density on gas transfer during HFV.

In other indirect support of Knopp, Solway and others, Fletcher and Epstein[89] concluded that facilitated diffusion did not play a critical role in HFOV because physiologic dead space calculated during HFOV in rabbits remained virtually unchanged through a frequency range from 1 to 22 Hz. However, Weinman et al.[85] reported a reduction of V_D during HFV, with the fall in V_D related to a decrease in V_T and Jonzon et al.[90] demonstrated a decrease in alveolar dead space during HFPPV at a frequency of only 100/min. They also reported that the dead space was reduced further with positive pressure end-expiratory pressure (PEEP).

When all the reports are examined carefully, and an attempt is made to eliminate reports which are based on data which might not be valid, it appears that the dependency on density-related transport mechanisms is not great. Physiologic dead space may decrease enough to accommodate gas exchange with smaller tidal volumes than might be expected, but it is very difficult to measure V_D accurately at high frequencies. Using these arguments, Chakrabarti et al.[91] believed it was unnecessary to evoke the theory of enhanced diffusion due to frequency per se during HFPPV or HFOV in a lung model they studied. Colgan et al.[92,93] also concluded that gas exchange during HFV can be explained by conventional concepts, and no benefit can be expected from frequencies greater than 200/min because of increased ventilation requirements. However, the reduction in physiological V_D which is proposed to be necessary when f is high and tidal volume is small (but ventilation still supports gas exchange) is difficult for many investigators to accept. Therefore, some other method of mixing in the airways, or some other way of reducing the effect of the anatomic space, would be welcomed.

Lehr[94] has proposed that the lungs are inflated asymmetrically, with some units as much as 180° out of phase. This principle was demonstrated with excised dog lungs photographed during HFOV under stroboscopic light. His ''disco lung'' appeared to undergo ''Pendelluft'' movement in which significantly different time constants (the product of resistance and compliance) for individual lung units permitted retrograde or intra-alveolar flow to equilibrate with slowly filling units from gas contained in those which have shorter time constants and are, therefore, filled more quickly. West and Hugh-Jones[75] also observed asynchronous air movement between different parts of the lung in their report on cardiac oscillations in the bronchi. Thus, a much smaller volume of gas can be spread out among more alveoli, reducing the effective dead space. However, many investigators would like some evidence that this can account for gas exchange during HFV where V_D/V_T can be as high as 4.0.*

Haselton and Scherer[95] proposed that oscillations can transfer gases in a bifurcating tube due to velocity profiles which change with the direction of flow. Over repeated cycles, a net flow forward (toward the branch) is observed in the center and a net flow backward (away from the branch) occurs at the edge of the tube, even though total bulk flow is zero. This could provide considerable movement of respiratory gases at high frequency in the multi-branching airway system as a result of such asymmetric velocity profiles. However, augmented airway mixing occurs in straight (nonbranching) tubes so bifurcations cannot provide the total explanation for the effectiveness of HFV.

The asymmetry of the airway permits some gas exchange in regions from airways whose anatomic dead space is less than the overall dead space (for instance, those near the hila). These alveoli could be adequately ventilated with tidal volumes well under dead space volume[3] so gas exchange can occur with $V_D/V_T > 1.0$ without invoking diffusion-related phenomena. Simon et al.[96] conjectured that inspiratory and expiratory airway impedances were different, and Goldstein and Mead[97] reported that absolute respiratory impedance was 14% greater during expiration than during inspiration at a driven frequency of 8.5 Hz. It is conceivable that these differences would permit an asymmetrical pattern of flow in at least some part of the airway, with streamline flow during inspiration (when the airway was larger) followed by turbulent flow during expiration (when velocity was higher). This would provide dissimilar velocity profiles, and, therefore, uneven mixing upstream and downstream.

* In Chapter 2 Wayne Mitzner dramatically demonstrates that effective dead space is, indeed, reduced by having at least some part of even small tidal volumes reach the alveoli. He demonstrates that HFV can work with small tidal volumes if there is a sufficiently large ''dispersion coefficient'', related to a diversity of effective path lengths or transit times for inspired air to get to the alveoli. He has, for the moment at least, not defined the determinants of the dispersion coefficient. That definition may go far toward clarifying *how* HFV works, and when it might not, and it may be what other investigators are woking on, even though they are calling it something else.

A somewhat unexpected finding has been reported by investigators who measured peripheral (alveolar) pressures and compared them with pressure at the mouth. Jackson et al.[98] predicted, on the basis of a computer model, that peripheral airway pressure was higher than in central airways during HFV at some frequencies. This observation supported similar observations by Keefe et al.[99] Simon et al.[96] also demonstrated that P_{aw} could underestimate P_{alv} at high frequencies, with greater differences observed at larger V_T and lower P_{aw}. They related the pressure differences to differences in inspiratory and expiratory gas-flow impedances. Beamer et al.[100] agreed that at high frequencies gas trapping could exist because of an increased expiratory impedance, which increases P_{alv} without affecting proximal P_{aw}. This may exert deleterious effects on patients with obstructive impairment if they are subjected to HFV. Sutton and Glass,[101] on the other hand, believed that having the peripheral pressure elevated over central airway pressure could reduce atelectasis, improve oxygenation, and increase FRC. Boynton et al.[62,102] carefully measured pressures at the airway opening and in the trachea of 11 neonates, and reported P_{tr} usually less than or equal to P_{aw} during HFOV or HFOV plus IMV. From this, it is evident that changes in geometry which induced the difference in impedance between inspiration and expiration must have occurred in smaller airways, probably those unsupported by cartilage.

Progress toward understanding the principle of HFV has been made as a result of the contributions of both clinical investigators and basic scientists in the field. Some workers, in their eagerness, depended on inadequately controlled studies, and others, in their enthusiasm, supported incompletely developed hypotheses. But the controversies which resulted have helped clarify the questions and contributed to the answers. Discussions at scientific meetings (either clinical or basic) have been vigorous and provocative, and they often sent the attendees back to their laboratories to challenge statements they heard (or, sometimes, only thought they heard). The fundamental question is still not completely settled: can physiologic dead space be reduced sufficiently by some process of "enhanced airway mixing" in regions of either laminar or turbulent flow to permit gas exchange to proceed with tidal volumes as small as perceived? Some investigators find no problem with accepting that concept, but others believe either that the *effective* tidal volume is larger than estimated, or that the *effective* dead space is smaller. Mitzner, in his chapter of this book, provides an argument which says that the latter is true.

Progress toward a better understanding of HFV will depend on continuing the dialogue. A more widespread clinical use of HFV will result from improvements in ventilators and from developing more reliable and extensive monitoring techniques. Techniques which introduce and control PEEP are being studied in ventilators for investigational use. The combination of HFV and IMV or periodic sighing breaths, previously recommended by only a few investigators, is now widely accepted and is being accommodated in new instrumentation systems. Periodic measurements of FRC, P_{alv}, and ventilation (both total and effective) still need to be simplified so they can be used routinely in clinical applications of HFV.

Some of the overly enthusiastic promises which accompanied early observations about HFV threatened its credibility and its survival. They have now given way to realistic statements and hard work to define the role of HFV in medicine. There are many reasons to believe that the technique will continue to be important, and that it will develop into a predictable, useful tool for assisted ventilation in clinical cases previously not treated effectively. There are also reasons to believe that the principles on which HFV is based will become more clear, so techniques can be developed to assure its application where it will be most effective.

REFERENCES

1. Froese, A. B., High frequency ventilation: current status, *Can. Anaesth. Soc. J.*, 31, S9, 1984.
2. Henderson, Y., Chillingsworth, F. P., and Whitney, J. L., The respiratory dead space, *Am. J. Physiol.*, 38, 1, 1915.
3. Briscoe, W. A., Forster, R. E., and Comroe, J. H., Jr., Alveolar ventilation at very low tidal volumes, *J. Appl. Physiol.*, 7, 27, 1954.
4. Duffner, L. R., Hamilton, L. H., and Schmitz, M. A., Effect of whole-body vertical vibration on respiration in human subjects, *J. Appl. Physiol.*, 17, 913, 1962.
5. Sjostrand, U., Review of the physiological rationale for and development of high frequency positive pressure ventilation, *Acta Anaesthesiol.*, Suppl. 64, 7, 1977.
6. Sjostrand, U., High frequency positive pressure ventilation: a review, *Crit. Care Med.*, 8, 345, 1980.
7. Sjostrand, U., Low-Compression high frequency positive pressure ventilation: a review, *Resuscitation*, 11, 183, 1984.
8. Draper, W. B. and Whitehead, R. W., Diffusion respiration in the dog anesthetized with Pentothal Sodium, *Anesthesiology*, 5, 262, 1944.
9. Lunkenheimer, P. P., Keller, H., Frank, I., Dickhut, H. H., and Fuhrman, C., Application of transtracheal pressure oscillations as a modification of "Diffusion Respiration", *Br. J. Anaesth.*, 44, 627, 1972.
10. Frank, I., Ising, H., and Keller, H., Intrapulmonaler Gasweehsel unter simulierter Apnoe durch transtrachealen, peridoischen intrathorakelen Druckwechsel, *Anaestheisist*, 22, 232, 1973.
11. Bohn, D. J., Butler, W., Froese, A. B., and Bryan, A. C., Ventilation by high frequency oscillation, *Fed. Proc.*, 38, 951, 1979.
12. Butler, W. J., Bohn, D. J., Bryan, A. C., and Forese, A. B., Ventilation by high frequency oscillation in humans, *Anesth. Analg.*, 59, 577, 1980.
13. Sanders, R. D., Two ventilating attachments for bronchoscopes, *Del. Med. J.*, 39, 170, 1967.
14. Klain, M. and Smith, R. B., High frequency percutaneous transtracheal jet ventilation, *Crit. Care Med.*, 5, 280, 1977.
15. Klain, M., Keszler, H., and Brader, E., High frequency jet ventilation in CPR, *Crit. Care Med.*, 9, 421, 1981.
16. Smith, R. B. and Klain, M., Experimental high frequency ventilation, in *International Anesthesiology Clinics: High Frequency Ventilation*, Vol. 21, Smith, R. B. and Sjostrand, V. H., Eds., Little Brown, Boston, 1983, 33.
17. Rouby, J. J., Fusciardi, J., Bourgain, J. L., and Viars, P., High frequency ventilation in postoperative respiratory failure: determinants of oxygenation, *Anesthesiology*, 59, 281, 1983.
18. Carlon, G. C., Klain, M., Kalla, R., Trunbull, A. D., and Kahn, R. C., High frequency positive-pressure ventilation: applications in acute respiratory failure, *Crit. Care Med.*, 7, 128, 1979.
19. Carlon, G. C., Howland, W. S., Klain, M., Goldiner, P. L., and Ray, C., Jr., High frequency positive ventilation for ventilatory support in patients with Broncho-Pleural Fistulas, *Crit. Care Med.*, 7, 128, 1979.
20. Gallagher, T. J., Klain, M., and Carlon, G. C., Present status of high frequency ventilation, *Crit. Care Med.*, 10, 613, 1982.
21. Meeuwis, H., Vaes, L., and Klain, M., Long-term high frequency jet ventilation in a 3-yr old child, *Crit. Care Med.*, 11, 309, 1981.
22. Sladen, A. and Klain, M., High frequency jet ventilation: a case report, *Thorax*, 37, 558, 1982.
23. Schuster, D. P., Klain, M., and Snyder, J. V., Comparison of high frequency jet ventilation to conventional ventilation during severe acute respiratory failure in humans, *Crit. Care Med.*, 10, 625, 1982.
24. Sladen, A., Guntpalli, K., Marquez, J., and Klain, M., High frequency jet ventilation in the postoperative period: a review of 100 patients, *Crit. Care Med.*, 12, 782, 1984.
25. Carlon, G. C., Howland, W. S., Groeger, J. S., Ray, C., Jr., and Miodownik, S., Role of high frequency jet ventilation in the management of respiratory failure, *Crit. Care Med.*, 12, 777, 1984.
26. Groeger, J. S., Carlon, G. C., Howland, W. S., Ray, C., Jr., and Miodownik, S., Experimental evaluation of high frequency jet ventilation, *Crit. Care Med.*, 12, 747, 1984.
27. Calkins, J. M., Waterson, C. K., Hameroff, S. R., Harris, T. R., and Jones, J. F., A simple flueric high frequency jet ventilator, *Anesth. Analg.*, 61, 138, 1982.
28. Rone, C. A., Pavlin, E. G., Cummings, C. W., and Weymuller, E. A., Studies in transtreacheal ventilation catheters, *Laryngoscope*, 92, 1259, 1982.
29. Carlon, G. C., Miodownik, S., Ray, C., Jr., and Kahn, R. C., Technical aspects and clinical implications of high frequency jet ventilation with a solenoid valve, *Crit. Care Med.*, 9, 47, 1981.
30. Davey, A. J., Lay, G. R., and Leigh, J. M., High frequency venturi jet ventilation, *Anaesthesia*, 37, 947, 1982.

31. Ramanthan, S., Sinha, K., Arismendy, J., Chaln, J., and Turndorf, H., Humidification and airway pressures during high frequency jet ventilation delivered through the suction-biopsy channel of a flexible bronchofiberscope, *Crit. Care Med.,* 12, 820, 1984.
32. Smith, R. B., Sjostrand, U., and Babinski, M. J., Technical considerations using high frequency positive pressure ventilation and high frequency jet ventilation, in *International Anesthesiology Clinics; High Frequency Ventilation,* Vol. 21, Smith, R. B. and Sjostrand, U. H., Eds., Little, Brown, Boston, 1983, 183.
33. Doyle, H. J., Napolitano, A. E., Lippman, H. R., Cooper, K. R., Duncan, J. S., Eakins, K., and Glauser, F., Different humidification systems for high frequency jet ventilation, *Crit. Care Med.,* 12, 815, 1984.
34. Ramanathan, S., Arismendy, J., Gandhi, S., Chalon, J., and Turndoff, H., Coaxial catheter for humidification during jet ventilation, *Anesth. Analg.,* 61, 689, 1982.
35. Ritz, R., Benson, M., and Bishop, M. J., Measuring gas leakage from bronchopleural fistulas during high frequency jet ventilation, *Crit. Care Med.,* 12, 836, 1984.
36. Quan, S. F., Calkins, J. M., Waterson, C. K., Conahan, T. J., Hameroff, S. R., and Otto, C. W., Airway movement in dogs during high frequency jet ventilation, *Crit. Care Med.,* 12, 452, 1984.
37. Ray, C., Jr., Miodownik, S., Carlon, G., Groeger, J., and Howland, W. S., Pneumatic-to-electric analog for high frequency jet ventilation of disrupted airways, *Crit. Care Med.,* 12, 711, 1984.
38. Sladen, A., Guntupalli, K., and Klain, M., High frequency jet ventilation vs. intermittent positive-pressure ventilation, *Crit. Care Med.,* 12, 788, 1984.
39. Lyons, D., Stenzler, A., Steinberg, H., Abramson, A., and Ruder, C., The airway mechanics of jet ventilation, *Otolaryngol. Head Neck Surg.,* 89, 364, 1981.
40. Hamilton, L. H., Londino, J. M., Linehan, J. H., and Neu, J., Pediatric endotracheal tube designed for high frequency ventilation, *Crit. Care Med.,* 12, 988, 1984.
41. Vourc'h, G., Fischler, M., Michon, F., Melchior, J. C., and Seigneu, R. F., High frequency jet ventilation vs. manual jet ventilation during bronchoscopy in patients with tracheo-bronchial stenosis, *Br. J. Anaesth.,* 55, 969, 1983.
42. Derderian, S. S., Rajagopal, K. R., Abbrecht, P. H., Bennet, L. L., Doblar, D. D., and Hunt, K. K., Jr., High frequency positive pressure ventilation in bilateral bronchopleural fistuale, *Crit. Care Med.,* 10, 119, 1982.
43. Schmale, T. J., Brown, M., and Brown, E. M., High frequency jet ventilation in a patient with sarcoidosis and bilateral bronchopleural fistuale, *J. Nat. Med. Assoc.,* 76, 193, 1984.
44. Seki, S., Goto, K., Kondo, T., Fukushima, Y., Konishi, H., and Kosaka, F., Gas exchange and facilitation of high frequency ventilation in intrathoracic surgery, *Ann. Thorac. Surg.,* 37, 491, 1984.
45. Smith, R. B., Hoff, B. H., Rosen, L., Wilson, E., and Swartzman, S., High frequency ventilation during pulmonary lobectomy, *Respir. Care,* 26, 437, 1981.
46. Hoff, B. H., Wilson, E., Smith, R. B., Bennet, E., and Philips, W., Intermittent positive pressure ventilation and high frequency ventilation in dogs with experimental bronchopleural fistulae, *Crit. Care Med.,* 11, 598, 1983.
47. Carlon, G. C., Griffin, J., Ray, C., Jr., Groeger, J. S., and Patrick, K., High frequency jet ventilation in experimental airway disruption, *Crit. Care Med.,* 11, 353, 1983.
48. Swartzman, S., Wilson, M. A., Hoff, B. A., Bunegin, L., Smith, R. B., and Sjostrand, U., Percutaneous transtracheal jet ventilation for cardiopulmonary resuscitation: evaluation of a new jet ventilator, *Crit. Care Med.,* 12, 8, 1984.
49. Harf, A., Bertrand, C., and Chang, H. K., Ventilation by high frequency oscillation of thorax or at trachea in rats, *J. Appl. Physiol.,* 56, 155, 1984.
50. Zidulka, A., Minami, H., Gross, D., Vartia, V., and Chang, H. K., Ventilation by high frequency chest wall compression in dogs with normal lungs, *Am. Rev. Respir. Dis.,* 127, 709, 1983.
51. Ward, H. E., Power, J. H. T., and Nicholas, T. E., High Frequency Oscillations via the pleural surface: an alternative mode of ventilation?, *J. Appl. Physiol.,* 54, 427, 1983.
52. Chang, H. K. and Harf, A., High frequency ventilation: a review, *Resp. Physiol.,* 57, 135, 1984.
53. Frantz, I. D., Stark, A. R., and Dorkin, H. L., Ventilation of infants at frequencies up to 1800/min, *Pediatr. Res.,* 14, 642, 1980.
54. Frantz, I. D., Werthammer, J., and Stark, A. R., High frequency ventilation in premature infants with lung disease; adequate gas exchange at low tracheal pressure, *Pediatrics,* 71, 483, 1983.
55. Bland, R. D., Kim, M. H., Light, M. J., Woodson, J. L., and Hodson, W. A., High frequency mechanical ventilation in severe hyaline membrane disease, *Crit. Care Med.,* 8, 275, 1980.
56. Jones, L. S., High frequency ventilation for immature infants, *Pediatrics,* 71, 280, 1983.
57. Truog, W. E., Standaert, T. A., Murphy, J. H., Woodrum, D. E., and Hodson, W. A., Effects of prolonged high frequency oscillation ventilation in premature primates with experimental hyaline membrane disease, *Am. Rev. Respir. Dis.,* 130, 76, 1984.

58. Bryan, C., Jobe, A. H., Ikegami, M., Jacobs, H. C., and Saramiento, A., High frequency oscillations vs. conventional ventilation of premature lambs, *Neonatology,* 33, 1982.
59. Carlo, W. A., Chatburn, R. L., Martin, R. J., Lough, M. D., Shivpuri, C. R., Anderson, J. V., and Fanaroff, A. A., Decrease in airway pressure during high frequency jet ventilation in infants with respiratory distress syndrome, *J. Pediatr.,* 104, 101, 1984.
60. Pokora, T., Bing, D., Mammel, M., and Boros, S., Neonatal high frequency jet ventilation, *Pediatrics,* 72, 27, 1983.
61. Neu, J., Hamilton, L. H., Linehan, J. H., Rich, M., Murkowski, K., Wilson, A., and Oechler, H., Long-term high frequency jet ventilation in neonates, *Crit. Care Med.,* 12, 833, 1984.
62. Boynton, B. R., Mannino, F. L., Davis, R. F., Kopotic, R. J., and Friederichsen, G., Combined high frequency oscillation ventilation and intermittent mandatory ventilation in critically ill neonates, *J. Pediatr.,* 105, 297, 1984.
63. Karl, S. R., Ballantine, T. V. N., and Snider, M. T., High frequency ventilation at rates of 375 to 1800/CPM in four neonates with congenital diaphragmatic hernia, *J. Pediatr. Surg.,* 18, 822, 1983.
64. DeLemos, R. A., Null, D. M., Jr., and Meredith, K. S., High frequency ventilation: panacea or problem?, *Pediatrics,* 69, 240, 1982.
65. Truog, W. E., Standaert, T. A., Murphy, J., Palmer, S., Woodrum, D. E., and Hodson, W. A., Effect of high frequency oscillation on gas exchange and pulmonary phospholipids in experimental RDS, *Am. Rev. Respir. Dis.,* 127, 585, 1983.
66. Bland, R. D. and Sedin, E. G., High frequency mechanical ventilation in the treatment of neonatal respiratory distress, in *International Anesthesiology Clinics; High Frequency Ventilation,* Vol. 21, Smith, R. B. and Sjostrand, U. H., Eds., Little, Brown, Boston, 1983, 125.
67. Thompson, W. K., Marchak, B. E., Froese, A. B., and Bryan, A. C., High frequency oscillation compared with standard ventilation in pulmonary injury model, *J. Appl. Physiol.,* 52, 543, 1982.
68. Calkins, J. M., Waterson, C. K., Hameroff, S. R., and Kanel, J., Jet pulse characteristics for high frequency jet ventilation in dogs, *Anesth. Analg.,* 61, 293, 1982.
69. Carlon, G. C., Ray, C., Jr., Miodowniks, S., Howland, W. S., Guy, Y., and Groeger, J. S., Physiologic implications of high frequency jet ventilation techniques, *Crit. Care Med.,* 11, 508, 1983.
70. Ahmann, P. A., Lazzara, A., Dykes, F. D., Schwartz, J. F., and Brann, A. W., Jr., Intraventricular hemorrhage: incidence and outcome, *Ann. Neurol.,* 4, 186, 1978.
71. Dykes, F. D., Ahmann, P. A., Lazzara, A., Brann, A. W., Jr., and Schwartz, J. F., Interventricular hemorrhage: an iatrogenic complication, *Ann. Neurol.,* 4, 187, 1978.
72. Raju, T. N., Braverman, B., Nadkarny, U., Kim, W. D., and Vidyasagar, D., Intracranial pressure and cardiac output remain stable during high frequency oscillation, *Crit. Care Med.,* 11, 856, 1983.
73. Toutant, S. M., Todd, M. M., Frummond, J. C., and Shapiro, H. M., Cerebral blood flow during high frequency ventilation in cats, *Crit. Care Med.,* 11, 712, 1983.
74. Grasberger, R. C., Spatz, E. L., Mortara, R. W., Ordia, J. I., and Yeston, N. S., Effect of high frequency ventilation vs. conventional ventilation on ICP in head-injured dogs, *J. Neurosurg.,* 60, 1214, 1984.
75. West, J. B. and Hugh-Jones, P., Pulsatile gas flow in bronchi caused by the heart beat, *J. Appl. Physiol.,* 16, 697, 1961.
76. Drechsler, D. M. and Ultman, J. S., Cardiogenic mixing in the pulmonary conducting airway of Man?, *Resp. Physiol.,* 56, 37, 1984.
77. Slutsky, A. S., Gas mixing by cardiogenic oscillations: a theoretical quantitative analysis, *J. Appl. Physiol.,* 51, 1287, 1981.
78. Slutsky, A. S., Drazen, J. M., Ingram, R. H., Jr., Kamm, R. D., Shapiro, A. H., Fredberg, J. J., Loring, S. H., and Lehr, J., Effective pulmonary ventilation with small volume oscillation at high frequency, *Science,* 209, 609, 1980.
79. Fredberg, J. J., Augmented diffusion in the airways can support pulmonary gas exchange, *J. Appl. Physiol.,* 49, 232, 1980.
80. Knopp, T. J., Kaethner, T., Meyer, M., Rehder, K., and Scheid, P., Gas mixing in the airways of dogs lungs during high frequency ventilation, *J. Appl. Physiol.,* 55, 1141, 1983.
81. Robertson, H. T., Coffey, R. L., Standaert, T. A., and Trugg, W. E., Respiratory and inert gas exchange during high frequency ventilation, *J. Appl. Physiol.,* 55, 1141, 1983.
82. Khoo, M. C. K., Slutsky, A. S., Drazen, J. M., Solway, J., Gavriely, N., and Kamm, R. D., Gas mixing during high frequency ventilation: an improved model, *J. App. Physiol.,* 57, 493, 1984.
83. Solway, J., Gavriely, N., Kamm, R. D., Drazen, J. M., Ingram, R. H., and Khoo, M. C. K., Intra-airway gas mixing during high frequency ventilation, *J. Appl. Physiol.,* 56, 343, 1984.
84. Goldstein, D., Slutsky, A. S., Ingram, R. H., Westerman, P., Venegas, J., and Drazen, J., CO2 elimination by high frequency ventilation (4—10 HZ) in normal subjects, *Am. Rev. Respir. Dis.,* 123, 251, 1981.
85. Weinmann, G. G., Mitzner, W., and Permutt, S., Physiological dead space during high frequency ventilation in dogs, *J. Appl. Physiol.,* 57, 881, 1984.

86. Solway, J., Gouriely, N., Slutsky, A. S., and Drazer, J. M., Effect of resident gas on CO_2 output during high frequency ventilation, *Fed. Proc.*, 42, 1350, 1983.
87. Goldman, L. J. and MacDonald, J. S., The role of resident gas on CO2 exchange during high frequency ventilation, *Anesthesiology*, 59, A495, 1983.
88. Brusasco, V., Knopp, T. J., and Rehder, K., Gas transport during high frequency ventilation, *J. Appl. Physiol.*, 55, 472, 1983.
89. Fletcher, P. R. and Epstein, R. A., Constancy of Physiological dead space during high frequency ventilation, *Resp. Physiol.*, 47, 39, 1984.
90. Jonzon, A., Rondio, Z., and Sedin, G., Alveolar dead space during high frequency positive pressure ventilation, *Br. J. Anesth.*, 55, 1133, 1983.
91. Chakrabarti, M. D., Loh, L., and Gilchrist, I., High frequency ventilation and gas diffusion, *Acta Anaesthesiol. Scand.*, 28, 544, 1984.
92. Colgan, F. J., Teneyck, L. G., and Sawa, T., Ventilation requirements during high frequency ventilation, *Crit. Care Med.*, 11, 173, 1983.
93. Colgan, F. J., Teneyck, L. G., and Sawa, T., Ventilatory requirements during high frequency ventilation in dogs, *Anesth. Analg.*, 61, 175, 1982.
94. Lehr, J., Circulating currents during high frequency ventilation, *Fed. Proc.*, 39, 576, 1980.
95. Haselton, F. R. and Scherer, P. W., Bronchial bifurcations and respiratory mass transport, *Science*, 208, 69, 1980.
96. Simon, B. A., Weinmann, G. G., and Mitzner, W., Mean airway pressure and alveolar pressure during high frequency ventilation, *J. Appl. Physiol.*, 57, 1069, 1984.
97. Goldstein, D. and Mead, J., Total respiratory impedance immediately after panting, *J. Appl. Physiol.*, 48, 1024, 1980.
98. Jackson, A. C., Tabrizi, M., Kotlikoff, M. I., and Voss, J. R., Airway pressures in asymmetrically branched airway model of dog respiratory system, *J. Appl. Physiol.*, 57, 1222, 1984.
99. Keefe, D., Glass, G., Castile, R., Frantz, I., Stark, A., and Fredberg, J. J., Alveolar pressure during high frequency oscillation in excised dog lungs, *Fed. Proc.*, 42, 763, 1983.
100. Beamer, W. C., Prough, D. S., Royster, R. L., Johnston, W. E., and Johnson, J. C., High frequency jet ventilation produces auto-PEEP, *Crit. Care Med.*, 12, 734, 1984.
101. Sutton, J. E. and Glass, D., Airway pressure gradient during high frequency ventilation, *Crit. Care Med.*, 12, 774, 1984.
102. Boynton, B. R., Mannino, F. L., Meathe, E. A., Kopotic, R. J., and Friederichsen, G., Airway pressure measurement during high frequency oscillatory ventilation, *Crit. Care Med.*, 12, 39, 1984.
103. Mitzner, W., Personal communications.

Chapter 2

HIGH FREQUENCY VENTILATION: WHY IT WORKS

Wayne Mitzner

TABLE OF CONTENTS

I. INTRODUCTION

The main purpose of this chapter is to attempt to provide some intuitive insight into how and why HFV works. An attempt will be made to avoid sophisticated fluid dynamics or engineering analysis in this chapter, since such analyses are unlikely to help provide insight for those unfamiliar with these mathematical approaches. A detailed and comprehensive review of the many different types of mechanisms proposed will also be avoided, since there are already several excellent such reviews in the literature.[5,7,13] In the present chapter an approach to understanding HFV is presented, which hopefully will provide a framework in which to view the various mechanisms catalogued in the more complete published reviews.

Since HFV is being discussed, perhaps the best place to start is with a definition of HFV. Considering the fact that there are so many investigators studying and using HFV, it is perhaps surprising that a general consensus on its definition has not been reached. Explicit in the very name high frequency ventilation is the suggestion that this mode of ventilation involves respiratory frequencies higher than normal. But since normal breathing frequencies vary within and among different species, using an absolute frequency range in the definition is of limited usefulness. Further complicating the situation is the fact that different technical modes of deliverying HFV within a given species usually use different frequency ranges. The FDA originally defined somewhat arbitrarily HFV as ventilation with rates exceeding 150 breaths/min. Smith[23] has suggested that high frequency oscillation applies to rates between 400 and 2400 breaths/min, HFJV applies to rates 100 to 400 breaths/min, and high frequency positive pressure ventilation applies to rates between 60 and 100 breaths/min. Recently, Drazen et al.[7] have defined HFV as ventilation at a rate greater than four times the normal resting breathing frequency. This latter definition might allow one to compare results among different species whose resting rates can vary over a four- or fivefold range.

For the purpose of the present discussion, HFV will not be defined by the rates used, but rather by the tidal volume (V_T). It is clear that as tidal volume gets smaller the breathing frequency must increase, but it is not the increased frequency itself which is of great interest. The original report of Bohn et al.[2] which stimulated so much interest in HFV claimed that they achieved normal blood gases at an estimated V_T of only 20% of the anatomic dead space. Had this report only described ventilation at 15 Hz with V_T's of say 110% of the dead space, there would hardly have been much interest, and such a report might have never even been written, let alone published.

Therefore, HFV is made unique by the possibility of providing adequate ventilation with V_T less than dead space. The fact that frequencies must be increased above normal to achieve this may be of technical importance, but it is of secondary theoretical interest. Thus, the remainder of this discussion will attempt to explain how ventilation with tidal volumes apparently insufficient to wash out completely the dead space can result in adequate gas exchange.

II. CONCEPTUAL MODEL

Before considering the mechanisms which explain gas exchange under conditions where the tidal volume is less than the dead space volume (V_D), it might be helpful to consider why the classical model is not adequate. Conventionally the lung is divided into an alveolar compartment of uniform gas concentration where gas exchange with the blood takes place by diffusion, and a dead space compartment in which no gas exchange occurs.[6] Steady state exchange is proportional to tidal volume minus dead space volume, and thus, there is *no* steady state gas exchange when the tidal volume is less than or equal to the volume of the dead space. This conclusion is based on the

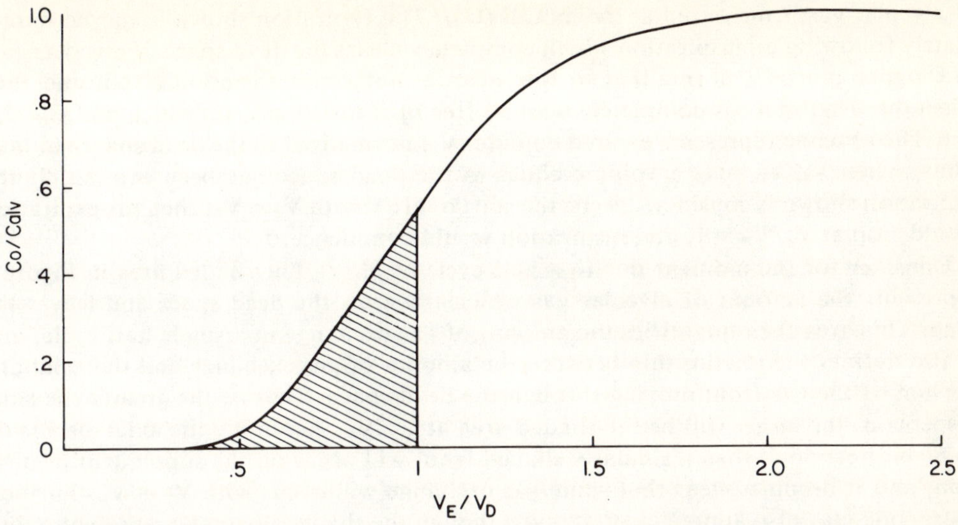

FIGURE 1. Hypothetical washout curve of alveolar gas, assuming no alveolar gas in the dead space at the start of expiration. The ordinate represents the gas concentration at the airway outlet (C_o) normalized to the mean alveolar concentration (C_{alv}). The abscissa represents expired volumed (V_E) normalized to the dead space volumed (V_D). The shaded area represents the amount of alveolar gas which traverses the dead space in a single expiration when $V_T = V_D$, (see text).

implicit assumption that during inspiration and expiration, gases traverse the dead space as a uniform or square front, where all gas molecules move with equal axial velocities. If such a simple model were correct, ventilation would clearly be impossible with tidal volume less than dead space, and thus, HFV as defined above, could not exist. However, the fact that all gas molecules do not traverse the dead space with uniform axial velocity has been known for many years, and this fact was used to account for early anecdotal reports of ventilation with tidal volumes less than anatomical dead space.[10] Furthermore, in the classical determination of dead space volume by the Fowler technique,[8] where the relation between the concentration of alveolar gas at the air outlet and volume expired is measured, the extent of the nonuniformity of velocities through the dead space is actually quantified. Thus within this context it is clear that some alveolar ventilation and gas exchange can take place with tidal volumes smaller than the dead space. Understanding how HFV works then becomes the task of understanding how alveolar and fresh gas are transported through the dead space at rates sufficient to provide the requisite gas exchange.

A. Gas Exchange when $V_T = V_D$

Let us now consider the special case of ventilation when V_T equals dead space volume. As already emphasized, if the front of gas moving through the dead space were perfectly square, there would be no alveolar ventilation. In the real lung, however, the front is not square,* and one might expect that the amount of alveolar ventilation would be very much dependent on how spread out the front of moving gas is. Throughout the remainder of this discussion, the term *axial dispersion* will be used to indicate this degree of spreading of the gas front along the tube axis.

Figure 1 shows a hypothetical washout curve of the lungs, where the concentration

* There are many reasons why the front might not be square and several proposed models of HFV are intimately concerned with these different reasons. For the purposes of this discussion, however, we need only be concerned with the fact that the front is not square and we ignore all the complexities of why this axial dispersion occurs.

of alveolar gas is measured at the mouth (C_O). The expiration shown is started immediately following an inspiration which completely clears the dead space of alveolar gas. The figure plots C_O normalized to the mean alveolar concentration (C_{alv}), and thus when the dead space is completely washed free of inspired gas, $C_O = C_{alv}$ and $C_O/C_{alv} = 1$. The abscissa represents expired volume (V_E) normalized to the dead space volume. Thus, when $V_E/V_D = 1$, a volume equal to the dead space has been expired. If the expiration shown is considered to be the start of HFV with $V_T = V_D$, then the expiration would stop at $V_E/V_D = 1$, and inspiration would commence.

Consider for the moment this first half cycle of HFV. The shaded area in Figure 1 represents the amount of alveolar gas which traverses the dead space and leaves the lung. This area then quantifies the amount of gas exchange in a single half cycle, and it also defines the relationship between the amount of gas exchange and the axial dispersion of the gas front moving through the dead space. That is, the greater the axial dispersion, the larger will be the shaded area at V_E/V_D. Assuming the axial dispersion to be bidirectional, then a similarly shaped front will occur on the subsequent inspiration, and it becomes clear that some gas exchange will occur with $V_T = V_D$. Furthermore, one may also appreciate that, even though the shaded area may represent only a small amount of alveolar gas, adequate gas exchange could be attained if the breathing frequency were made sufficiently high.

In the actual application of HFV with $V_T = V_D$, there will be an even greater gas exchange than that which might be predicted on the basis of the shaded area of Figure 1. This area does, indeed, represent the amount of direct transference of alveolar gas through the dead space, but after repeated ventilatory cycles, the dead space is not cleared of all alveolar gas during the inspiratory half cycle (which *was* the initial condition for the expiration shown in Figure 1). Therefore, during expiration in a steady state, the amount of alveolar gas which leaves will be equal to the shaded area plus a substantial portion of alveolar gas left in the dead space from the previous breaths. Quantitatively, this increase in steady state gas exchange compared to that for a single initial breath as described above has been estimated to be as much as 46%.[18]

B. Gas Exchange when V_T is less than V_D

From the above discussion, it may already be apparent that it is not necessary to have $V_T = V_D$ to support gas exchange. For the degree of axial dispersion of the gas front shown in Figure 1, it is clear that there would be some direct transference of alveolar gas when V_T is greater than about one third V_D since this is where the shaded area begins on the abscissa. For V_T less than one third V_D no alveolar gas would transit the dead space during the first expiration. However, if the flow velocity profile were not *completely* reversible, after the subsequent inspiration there would be some alveolar gas retained in the dead space. During the following expiration, this residual alveolar gas would be further transported toward the mouth. Once again, if this process were repeated frequently enough, it is conceivable that adequate alveolar ventilation could be maintained.

To analyze quantitatively the amount of gas exchange and the ventilatory frequency required to maintain it, one needs to have an index of the nonsquareness of the gas front moving through the dead space. One measure of this axial dispersion is the distribution function of transit times through the dead space. Those molecules of gas with the highest velocity will have the shortest transit time and will be manifested in the initial upslope of the washout curve in Figure 1. If the distribution of transit times is very broad, then a larger fraction of the gas will move through the dead space very quickly, and this would be expected to allow ventilation with smaller tidal volumes. Thus, the broader the transit time distribution, the better will ventilation be, everything else being equal. Statistically, the broadness of a distribution function is expressed by

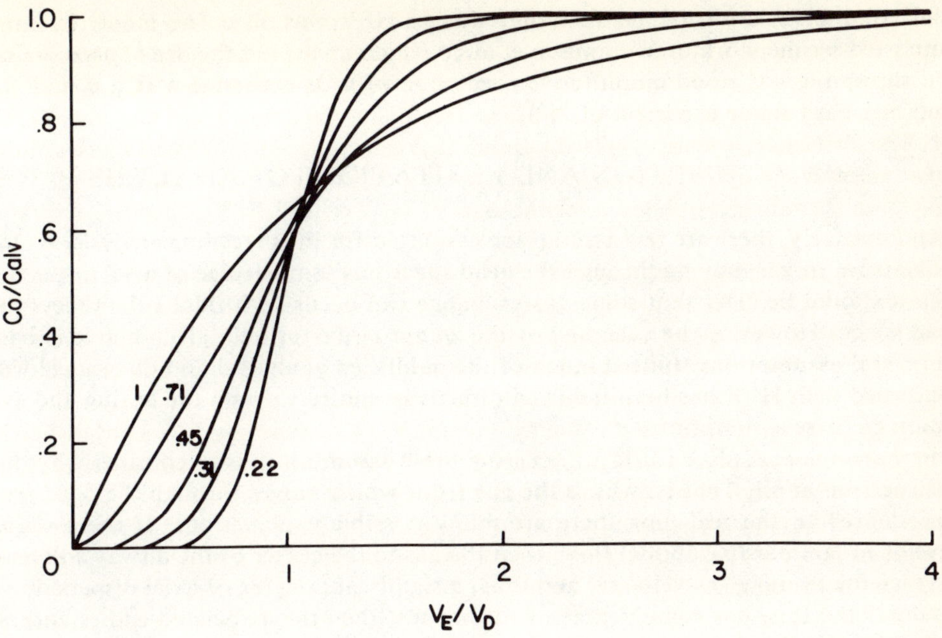

FIGURE 2. Influence of the degree of axial dispersion in the dead space on the expired concentration profile measured at the airway outlet (C_o). C_o is plotted normalized to the mean alveolar concentration (C_{alv}). The abscissa represents expired volume (V_E) normalized to dead space volume (V_D). The numbers associated with each curve represent different dispersion coefficients.

the standard deviation divided by the mean. For transit times, the symbol for the coefficient of dispersion is ($\sigma_t/\bar{t}$), where $\bar{t}$ = mean transit time and σ_t is the standard deviation of transit times. Figure 2 shows how the washout curve of Figure 1 would change with different dispersion coefficients. The curve in Figure 1 represents a $\sigma_t/\bar{t}$ of 0.33.

The general solution describing the quantitative relationship between gas exchange, ventilatory rate (f), tidal and dead space volumes (V_T and V_D) and the average coefficient of axial dispersion between inspiration and expiration ($\sigma_t/\bar{t}$) has been recently derived.[18] This solution (adapted for the special case of CO_2 exchange, $\dot{V}CO_2$) is given by the formula:

$$\dot{V}CO_2 = 0.6\,(\sigma_t/\bar{t})fV_D(V_T/V_D)^P\,F_ACO_2$$

where F_ACO_2 = alveolar CO_2 fraction and P = exponent to which tidal volume is raised.

It was also shown that P varies inversely with the square root of the coefficient of dispersion, and the formula for P is $P = 1 + 0.7\sqrt{\sigma_t/\bar{t}}$. In considering the above formula for $\dot{V}CO_2$, it is clear that the coefficient of dispersion plays a major role in determining how good gas exchange will be during HFV. Not only does $\sigma_t/\bar{t}$ appear in the equation as a direct multiplier, but it also determines the sensitivity of gas exchange to variations in tidal volume.

The coefficient of dispersion of transit times has not been measured directly during HFV. However, it has been calculated directly from the N_2 washout during a Fowler dead space determination.[18] Such curves typically show a dispersion coefficient of about 30%, and according to the above formula, if such a dispersion were obtained during HFV, the exponent, P, to which volume is raised would be slightly greater than 2.

Support for this analysis comes from recent studies[12,14,17,24] which reported that the tidal volume variation of gas exchange during HFV was V_T^2. The model is further supported by the work of Weinmann et al.,[25] which measured the dead space in dogs, and showed a very good quantitative prediction of CO_2 exchange with a $\sigma_t/\bar{t}$ of 0.32 (and hence a volume exponent of 2.2).

III. ASSUMPTION AND LIMITATIONS OF ANALYSIS

Qualitatively, there are few assumptions required for the preceding analysis. As long as the front of gas moving through the dead space has some degree of axial dispersion, then it should be clear that some gas exchange can occur with tidal volume less than dead space. However, the accuracy of the *quantitative* formula given above is based on several assumptions. Indeed much of the published analytical and theoretical work concerned with HFV has been involved directly or indirectly with the testing and evaluation of these assumptions.

Perhaps the best place to start discussing these assumptions is to consider why there is dispersion at all. That is, why is the gas front which moves through the dead space not square? In the real lung there are many possible explanations. If there is fully developed laminar (parabolic) flow, then the gas in the center of the airway will travel at twice the average gas velocity, and thus, a significant degree of axial dispersion will result. If the flow has some degree of turbulence, then the associated eddies and random motion will still cause some gas to penetrate the dead space faster, and some gas to penetrate it slower, than the mean gas transit time.

Also, in the lung, the distances between alveoli and the trachea are not constant, and thus, there will be some short and some long airway path lengths. This distribution of path lengths could lead to a distribution of transit times based solely on the different alveolar distances. This concept forms the basis of the "nearby alveolus" hypothesis described by Drazen et al.,[7] and analyzed in detail by Kamm et al.[13] Although there is no question that there are widely varying path lengths in the lung, the distribution of transit times through these varying paths has not been well studied. For example, in the extreme, if the velocities varied directly with path length (though such a mechanism is not easy to imagine), then the transit times would not vary, and the gas front through the airway tree could still be square.

The above quantitative analysis for small tidal volumes is based on the assumption that the flow pattern on expiration is not precisely reversed on the subsequent inspiration. There are several good reason to expect that flow streamlines are not the same on inspiration and expiration, and, indeed, they would only be reversible if the flow were always completely parabolic. To the extent that there is turbulence caused either by the high Reynold's numbers during HFV or by the flow distortion resulting from the airway bifurcations, the flow would not be reversible. Additionally, Schroter and Sudlow[20] have measured significantly different flow velocity profiles during inspiration and expiration in a branched airway model. Scherer and Haselton[19] have proposed that this flow asymmetry would lead to gas transport with tidal volumes smaller than the dead space, but they did not present a quantitative estimate of the magnitude of gas exchange.

It is worth emphasizing that the requirement that flow streamlines not be precisely reversed between inspiration and expiration is only really required for V_T *less than about* one third V_D (i.e., for the lung which gives rise to Figure 1). For V_T in the range where HFV is normally applied, there is a significant amount of direct gas transfer during a single breath. Thus, even if flow were completely reversible, the gas which already traversed the dead space could never be recovered and some gas exchange would still occur.

Another assumption on which the quantitative equation is based is that the dispersion coefficient of the transit time distribution is relatively insensitive to variation in flow. This is perhaps the weakest assumption, since there are some theoretical reasons to expect that the nature of the flow would influence the degree of dispersion. In the extreme, pure laminar, parabolic flow would have a different dispersion coefficient than would pure turbulent flow. However, flows in the real lung over the range between normal ventilation and HFV are neither purely laminar nor purely turbulent, and in this broad transitional flow range, it is theoretically possible to have little variation in the dispersion coefficient. That is, since the dispersion coefficient is expected to increase with increasing Reynolds number when the flow is laminar and to decrease with increasing Reynold's number when the flow is turbulent,[16] there must be a range where the dispersion coefficient is not changing greatly. That the range might indeed encompass normal and HFV flow rates is suggested by what little experimental evidence there is. Bouhuys[4] showed no difference for N_2 washout curves done at different expiratory flow rates. Indirect evidence was provided by Mitzner and Permutt,[17] who directly measured the dispersion coefficient in a long straight tube at a low steady flow rate. They then showed that this measured value gave a good quantitative prediction of the gas transport through this same tube during HFV with oscillatory volumes much less than the volume of the tube. Likewise, Weinmann et al.[25] showed that the magnitude of gas exchange during HFV in dogs could be predicted, based on the dispersion coefficient measured by Bouhuys during a conventional N_2 washout. Further evidence that the dispersion coefficient is flow insensitive comes from work with indicator dilution studies in the vascular system. Bassingthwaighte[1] has shown a constant dispersion coefficient over a range of flows in the transition region between laminar and turbulent flow.

IV. CONCLUSION

The model proposed here takes a global view of the whole gas transport process. It assumes only that the front of gas moving through the dead space is not square and that the flow streamlines are not reversible. The quantification of this nonsquareness by the dispersion coefficient, $\sigma_t/\bar{t}$, can be used to derive a quantitative prediction of the amount of gas exchange. Reasons for the dispersion are not relevant to this interpretation of HFV, but if such reasons were better understood, it would provide a more thorough picture. There have been many other models of HFV which have focused on the effects of airway geometry and the physical nature of flow in the airway[9,11,13,19,21,22] and the results of such studies may be used to characterize the underlying mechanisms providing the overall axial dispersion. A detailed discussion of the results of each of these models in relation to the present model is beyond the scope of this chapter.

In summary, the preceding qualitative model and quantitative equation is based on the existence of axial dispersion in the dead space, which is demonstrated during an ordinary Fowler determination of dead space. Based on such an observation, that is, with no greater degree of dispersion than has been observed for many years, it should have been no surprise that HFV would be compatible with adequate gas exchange. Yet nearly everyone, including the present author, was initially surprised. Perhaps one reason for this lack of perception is that it was not immediately apparent how the degree of dispersion demonstrated during an ordinary Fowler determination of dead space could be used to quantify the magnitude of gas exchange that would be expected during HFV. The model outlined above and analyzed in detail elsewhere[18] allows one to make such a quantification.

REFERENCES

1. Bassingthwaighte, J. B., Relative dispersion: a characterizing feature of specific vascular beds, *Anesth. Analg.*, 56, 72, 1977.
2. Bohn, D. J., Miyasaka, K., Marchak, B. E., Thompson, W. K., Froese, A. B., and Bryan, A. C., Ventilation by high-frequency oscillation, *J. Appl. Physiol.*, 48, 710, 1980.
3. Bouhuys, A., Respiratory dead space, in *Handbook of Physiology*, Vol. 1, Fenn W. O., and Rahn, H., Eds., American Physiology Society, Washington, D.C., 1964, 696.
4. Bouhuys, A., The anatomical dead space, in *Breathing*, Grune & Stratton, New York, 1974, 42.
5. Chang, H. K., Mechanisms of gas transport during ventilation by high frequency oscillation, *J. Appl. Physiol.*, 56, 553, 1984.
6. Comroe, J. H., Jr., Forster, R. E., DuBois, A. B., Briscoe, W. A., and Carlsen, E., *The Lung*, 2nd ed., Year Book, Chicago, 1962.
7. Drazen, J. M., Kamm, R. D., and Slutsky, A. S., High frequency ventilation, *Physiol. Rev.*, 64, 505, 1984.
8. Fowler, W. S., Lung function studies. II. The respiratory dead space, *Am. J. Physiol.*, 154, 405, 1948.
9. Fredberg, J. J., Augmented diffusion in the airways can support pulmonary gas exchange, *J. Appl. Physiol.*, 49, 232, 1980.
10. Henderson, Y., Chillingsworth, F. P., and Whitney, J. L., The respiratory dead space, *Am. J. Physiol.*, 38, 1, 1915.
11. Isabey, D., Harf, A., and Chang, H. K., Alveolar ventilation during high-frequency oscillation: core dead space concept, *J. Appl. Physiol.*, 56, 700, 1984.
12. Jaeger, M. J., Banner, M., and Gallager, J., Alveolar ventilation in high frequency studies, *Fed. Proc.*, 42 (Abstr.), 1351, 1983.
13. Kamm, R. D., Slutsky, A. S., and Drazen, J. M., High frequency ventilation, *CRC Crit. Rev., Biomed. Eng.*, 9, 347, 1984.
14. Kamm, R. D., Collins, J. M., Joshi, C. H., Greiner, M., and Shapiro, A. H., Axial dispersion of a passive contaminant in oscillatory flow, *Proc. Am. Conf. Eng. Med. Biol.*, 35, 23, 1982.
15. Khoo, M. C., Slutsky, A. S., Drazen, J. M., Solway, J., Gavriely, N., and Kamm, R. D., Gas mixing during high frequency ventilation: an improved model, *J. Appl. Physiol.*, 57, 493, 1984.
16. Levenspiel, O., Non-ideal flow, in *Chemical Reaction Engineering*, John Wiley & Sons, New York, 1962, 242.
17. Mitzner, W. and Permutt, S., High frequency ventilation: theoretical principles and experimental validation, *Am. Biomed. Eng.*, in press, 1985.
18. Permutt, S., Mitzner, W., and Weinmann, G. G., A model of gas transport during high frequency ventilation, *J. Appl. Physiol.*, in press, 1985.
19. Scherer, P. W. and Haselton, F. R., Convective exchange in oscillatory flow through bronchial-tree models, *J. Appl. Physiol.*, 53, 1022, 1982.
20. Schroter, R. C. and Sudlow, M. F., Flow patterns in models of the human bronchial airways, *Respir. Physiol.*, 7, 341, 1969.
21. Slutsky, A. S., Drazen, J. M., Ingram, R. H., Jr., Kamm, R. D., Shapiro, A. H., Fredberg, J. J., Loring, S. H., and Lehr, J., Effective pulmonary ventilation with small volume oscillations at high frequency, *Science*, 209, 609, 1980.
22. Slutsky, A. S., Kamm, R. D., Rossing, T. H., Loring, S. H., Lehr, J., Shapiro, A. H., Ingram, R. H., Jr., and Drazen, J. M., Effects of frequency, tidal volume and lung volume on CO_2 elimination in dogs by high frequency (2—30 Hz), low tidal volume ventilation, *J. Clin. Invest.*, 68, 1475, 1981.
23. Smith, R. B., Ventilation at high respiratory frequencies, *Anesthesia*, 37, 1011, 1982.
24. Tarbell, J. M., Ultman, J. S., and Durlofsky, L., Oscillatory dispersion in a branching tube network, *J. Biomech. Eng.*, 104, 338, 1982.
25. Weinmann, G. G., Mitzner, W., and Permutt, S., Physiologic dead space during high frequency ventilation in dogs, *J. Appl. Physiol.*, 57, 881, 1984.

Chapter 3

PULMONARY GAS EXCHANGE

Peter D. Wagner

TABLE OF CONTENTS

I. INTRODUCTION

The recently rediscovered phenomenon of HFV has interested a variety of research workers with diverse areas of expertise including physics, engineering, bioengineering, physiology, and clinical medicine. In each of these disciplines, major challenges are posed by rapid delivery of small gas volumes to the lungs, but the problems are all ultimately directed toward the common goal of safe maintenance of pulmonary gas exchange. This diversity makes it difficult to outline what to cover in a review on gas exchange, since almost every aspect of HFV is more or less directly connected to the way in which gas exchange occurs. Moreover, there must be some overlap between this chapter and most others in this book, for the same reasons. However, this chapter will attempt to focus just on what is known about gas exchange and will not attempt to deal with even closely associated issues that are better treated elsewhere in this book. For example, the fundamental physical processes involved in transporting gas molecules between the airway opening and the alveolar blood:gas barrier are central to the concept of gas exchange, yet remain largely beyond the scope of this chapter in terms of a critical evaluation from the biophysical standpoint. So, too, are lengthy analyses of clinical experience with HFV. While such studies pay attention to gas exchange, they also describe how the modality may or may not damage the lungs in the short or, especially, long term. Such studies will be addressed herein only insofar as gas exchange issues are important.

When one reads the exponentially increasing numbers of papers concerned with gas exchange during HFV (Figure 1), one is struck by the relatively small number of different objectives. In other words, papers fall into one of only a few major categories, and this suggests a natural way to organize the wealth of published information for this chapter. Specifically, there seems to be:

1. Demonstrations of feasibility of HFV in normal or diseased lungs of animals or man
2. Clinical anecdotes and case histories of patients demonstrating advantages and/or disadvantages of HFV in special situations
3. Comparisons of the efficacy of HFV and conventional mechanical ventilation in sustaining gas exchange in normal or diseased lungs or animals or man
4. Studies attempting to define physical processes (mechanisms) important in the maintenance of gas exchange during HFV

This chapter will deal with each of these major topics. Difficulties in reaching simple and useful conclusions are expected, however, because of: (1) the tremendous range of pulmonary structure and function encountered (species from rats to man; ages from neonate to adult; pathologies from none to terminal respiratory failure of several etiologies); and (2) the many types of high frequency ventilator hardware available and, for any one such hardware type, the multiple ways in which any two users differ in their application of the modality. As noted constantly throughout this book, one must deal with HFPPV, HFJV, HFOV, and HFCWC. Within each, there are many operational parameters that can be varied; parameters related to time (frequency); volume (stroke volume); pressures and flows, and also within each type of ventilation there exist sometimes substantial variations in hardware design.

These complexities notwithstanding, an attempt will now be made to pull together the alarming profusion of experimental work in this area to better understand pulmonary gas exchange during HFV.

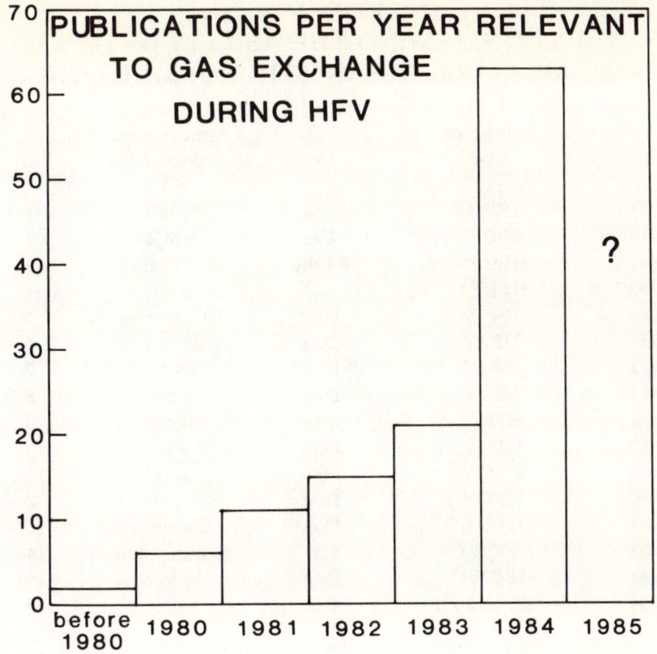

FIGURE 1. Number of publications that refer to pulmonary gas exchange during HFV of any type prior to 1980, and in each year subsequently. Note the large increase between 1983 and 1984. Undoubtedly, many new papers will be published in 1985. The point is that the field of HFV is in a stage of rapid expansion, and, as a result, the conclusions reached in this chapter may well have to be modified in the future.

II. FEASIBILITY OF MAINTENANCE OF GAS EXCHANGE BY HIGH FREQUENCY IN NORMAL LUNGS

There is abundant evidence, and no disagreement, that pulmonary gas exchange can be maintained under steady state conditions in normal animals and man without the development of CO_2 retention or hypoxemia. Table 1 shows a summary of publications documenting the ability to sustain gas exchange under normal conditions, and indicates both the type of high frequency ventilator and the species. In every case, the parameters of the ventilator could be adjusted to maintain arterial blood gas concentrations in the normal range for periods sufficiently long to be considered steady-state, and thus capable of sustaining metabolic needs. Furthermore, in normal animals and man, such conditions were not associated with particular negative side effects (except for mucosal inflammation near the tip of the jet in HFJV) as long as some obvious precautions were taken. For example, since a feature common to all forms of HFV is the to-and-fro movement of large volumes of gas in the upper airways, adequate humidification was early recognized to be important.[17,18] Without it, upper airway mucosal damage from drying became evident.[17] Avoidance of too high mean airway pressures has been a tacit operational guideline to the safe use of HFV to avoid parenchymal damage from over-inflation, and more will be said about this later. Histologic studies of lung parenchyma and airway epithelium, of markers of the surfactant system (type II alveolar epithelial cells, the alveolar lining layer) have consistently revealed no damage from carefully applied forms of HFPPV[19,20] and HFJV[21] used for periods of 2 to 24 hr. However, both anecdotal and systematic evidence exists documenting the en-

Table 1
STUDIES CONFIRMING THE ABILITY OF HFV TO MAINTAIN GAS EXCHANGE IN NORMAL LUNGS

Year	Ventilator type	Species	Approximate duration of HFV	Ref.
1971	HFPPV	Dog	20 min	1
1973	HFPPV	Cat	6 min	2
1982	HFPPV	Rabbit	10—15 min	3
1983	HFPPV	Cat	10 min	4
1984	HFPPV	Dog	20—30 min	5
1977	HFJV	Dog	20 min	6
1981	HFJV	Dog	24 hr	7
1984	HFJV	Dog	15 min	8
1972	HFOV	Dog	40 min	9
1980	HFOV	Dog	5 hr	10
1980	HFOV	Man	1 hr	11
1983	HFOV	Dog	15 min	12
1983	HFOV	Dog	36 hr	13
1983	HFCWC	Cat	30 min—6 hr	14
1983	HFCWC	Dog	30 min	15
1984	HFCWC and HFOV	Rat	5 min	16

hanced production of airway luminal mucus during HFV,[22] which may interfere with pulmonary gas exchange. Finally, a single report documents the appearance of small amounts of pleural fluid transudates during HFOV.[13] The authors speculate that the reason may be lack of tidal lung volume changes that are normally thought to enhance pulmonary lymph flow, but both the mechanisms and significance of this observation remain to be established.

III. FEASIBILITY OF MAINTENANCE OF GAS EXCHANGE BY HFV IN DISEASED LUNGS

Basically similar conclusions have been reached in animal models of disease and in many studies of patients with lung disease. Thus, ventilation by HFV can be successfully applied, in terms of gas exchange, in a majority of cases, by suitable choice of ventilator settings. When HFV has failed, it seems reasonable to conclude that conventional mechanical ventilation (CMV) was also insufficient, and the degree of pulmonary disease was simply too great to permit adequate ventilation by any means. Most of the studies that document feasibility of HFV in animal models of disease formally compared HFV to CMV. Accordingly, these are discussed in the subsequent section at some length, and this section will briefly summarize feasibility demonstrations of HFV in disease, mostly in patients requiring ventilatory support.

Table 2 lists the publications that deal primarily with documenting feasibility of sustaining gas exchange in disease. In oleic acid-induced pulmonary edema in rabbits, Wright et al.[38] showed in 1981 that adequate gas exchange could be maintained by HFOV at several combinations of MAP, fresh gas bias flow rate, oscillator stroke volume and frequency. It is unfortunate that neither lung volume nor cardiovascular data were obtainied, since it is likely that the effects of increasing each of the above HFOV parameters may well be mediated by a common mechanism, namely, lung volume recruitment. It would have been informative to see if the data obtained by varying one variable at a time would produce a single PaO_2-lung volume relationship, as suggested by subsequent studies discussed in the following section.

Sladen et al.[30] showed (in a series of 100 post-operative patients) that adequate ven-

Table 2
STUDIES CONFIRMING THE ABILITY OF HFV TO MAINTAIN GAS EXCHANGE IN DISEASED LUNGS

Year	Ventilator type	Situation species/or pathology/No. of subjects	Approximate duration of HFV	Ref.
1980	HFPPV	Human neonate/RDS/24	1—267 days	23
1983	HFPPV	Human neonate/RDS/15	1 hr	24
1984	HFPPV	Human adult/flail chest/2	3—4 days	25
1984	HFPPV	Human neonate/RDS/25	1—10 days	26
1984	HFPPV	Human adult/endoscopy/600	1 hr	27
1981	HFJV	Human adult/edema/1	days	28
1983	HFJV	Human adult/pneumonia/2	12—18 hr	29
1984	HFJV	Human adult/postoperative/100	1—21 days	30
1984	HFJV	Human adult/surgery for CA lung/12	Duration of surgery	31
1984	HFJV	Human adult/thoracic surgery/16	Duration of surgery	32
1984	HFJV	Human adult/respiratory weaning/9	24—192 hr	33
1984	HFJV	Human adult/ARDS/1	12 hr	34
1984	HFJV	Human adult/pneumonia/1	73 days	35
1984	HFJV	Human neonate/RDS/2	1 week	36
1984	HFJV	Human adult/atelectasis/1	3 days	37
1981	HFOV	Rabbit/oleic acid/11	20 min	38
1981	HFOV	Human neonate/RDS/8	1—10 hr	39
1984	HFOV	Human neonate/respiratory failure/12	6—192 hr	40

tilation and gas exchange could generally be obtained by using HFJV. This was found to be the case in all but two patients, and, in particular, 15 patients with respiratory failure were maintained for up to 21 days on HFJV. There were no reports of complications, and this, together with the high success rate, was encouraging. There was some evidence of cardiovascular depression at high airway pressures.

Marchak and co-workers[39] in 1981 reported on the use of HFOV in 8 neonates with respiratory distress. Arterial PO_2 was maintained at about 60 torr with a FIO_2 of about 0.40, compared to CMV where a similar arterial PO_2 required an FIO_2 of 0.66. In this study, HFOV was applied for 1 to 4 hr without apparent complications, either acutely or at a later follow-up some months later. Oxygenation was tightly related linearly to MAP, and thus presumably to lung volume.[38]

Eyal et al.[26] also reached positive conclusions in 25 neonates with severe respiratory distress, citing good survival and gas exchange, and low incidence of complications using HFPPV.

In 1980 Bland and co-workers[23] reported the effective use of HFPPV in 24 neonates with respiratory distress. While effective gas exchange was generally achievable, no measurement of airway pressures, lung volumes or cardiac output are given, making it difficult to deduce anything more than feasibility of HFPPV from the study. In the 24 infants, 29 serious complications were observed but without a control population one cannot clearly infer the role of HFPPV in the genesis of these problems. Boynton and co-workers[40] attempted HFOV in 12 neonates who could not be adequately ventilated by CMV. Most had a severe air leak, and under these circumstances, gas exchange improvement was noted, with survival of 8 of the 12 patients.

Seki et al.[31] and Scheck and Mallios[27] studied the efficacy of HFV in patients undergoing thoracic or upper airway surgery respectively, and reached positive conclusions. In essence, adequate gas exchange could be achieved while facilitating conduct of surgery due to less movement of the lungs and airways and better surgical access. Similar conclusions were reached by Mutz et al.[32] Klain et al.[33] further showed that in some cases HFJV permitted ventilator-dependent patients to be weaned from their ventilator, when the more usual approach of weaning by IMV had apparently failed. It is of interest that arterial PO_2 and PCO_2 were no different on CMV prior to HFJV than after 1 to 2 hr of HFJV, yet weaning was successful. The explanation for this is not apparent, nor is the role of HFV as a facilitating strategy in weaning in general. It is an area worthy of more study.

In another special situation, that of pre-existing barotrauma in infants, Frantz et al.[24] showed that better ventilation and gas exchange was observed during HFV.

Thus, in several settings of special interest, it has been demonstrated that adequate gas exchange can be obtained by HFV with apparent advantages over CMV and possibly no increase in deleterious side effects. However, all of these are uncontrolled studies and caution should be exercised before safety and efficacy are assumed to be satisfactory.

Finally, a number of case reports document the ability of HFV to maintain gas exchange, as listed in Table 2. These reports suggest improved mucociliary transport of secretions,[29] special advantages for the patient with flail chest,[25] less cardiovascular depression,[34] and special advantages in patients with bronchopleural fistulae[35] and with unilateral lung disease.[37] These results must be interpreted with even more caution than those described earlier in this section where measurements were made on groups of patients. Without a clear understanding of changes in lung volume and cardiovascular function, it is impossible to properly judge the benefit in each case. Probably, the case reports should form the basis of questions that might be answerable by controlled studies of a number of patients in each of the special circumstances particular to each report.

A. Summary of Feasibility Studies in Disease

Reports abound documenting adequacy of several forms of HFV in terms of ventilatory support and adequate gas exchange (Table 2). Such reports clearly indicate the need for well-controlled prospective comparisons of CMV and HFV, but should not themselves be taken as proof that HFV represents a complication-free major advance in ventilation of critically ill patients. In fact, as presented in the next section, such controlled comparative studies have all failed to show that, for general ventilatory support of patients in the ICU, gas exchange with HFV is any better than that with properly matched CMV.

IV. COMPARISONS BETWEEN HFV AND CONVENTIONAL VENTILATION IN NORMAL AND DISEASED LUNGS

The preceding section presented three conclusions:

1. Several types of HFV can maintain gas exchange in normal and diseased lungs for extended periods of time.
2. This can be achieved without apparent functional or structural complications or negative side effects if HFV is used with care.
3. There is definite potential for serious complications if HFV is not adequately set up and monitored.

The most likely of these are parenchymal disruption from sudden high distending pressures in the event of hardware malfunction; large airway mucosal damage, especially from HFVJ, and in particular, if humidification of inspired gas is inadequate; and finally, the consequences of increased airway luminal secretions, noted both anecdotally in patients, and more formally in experimental work.

Such a combination of potentially positive and negative effects has led to a considerable body of work attempting to compare the relative efficacy and safety of various forms of HFV to CMV. In other words, following demonstration of feasibility, the next major issue has been whether HFV has any special benefits compared to CMV.

Before summarizing such comparisons pertaining to gas exchange, it is worth addressing two issues that pervade the literature concerning this subject: (1) virtually every publication hypothesizes that the major potential benefits of HFV for general ventilatory support (i.e., in contrast to special situations such as bronchopleural fistula and thoracic surgery) are in reduced cardiovascular depression and lower incidence of pulmonary barotrauma. These hypotheses are founded on the premise that equivalent gas exchange will occur at lower "peak pressures" and perhaps at lower "mean airway pressures," and, therefore by presumption, at lower average alveolar pressures than during CMV. This is a critical concept in the rationale of HFV generally, not just in terms of gas exchange, and the following literature analysis will attempt to address the validity of this hypothesis. (2) Comparisons of HFV and CMV require some way of defining equivalence in order to reach conclusions on relative efficacy. Ultimately, the real yardstick for measuring the utility of HFV vs. CMV must be long term clinical outcome, but currently this is not generally possible. Most studies, therefore, have resorted to the tactic of matching one or more variable between CMV and HFV. The most common approach appears to have been to adjust the HFV parameters to match arterial PCO_2 and mean airway pressure (averaged over time). Then, the principal variables of comparative interest are indicators of arterial oxygenation, cardiovascular function and, sometimes, pulmonary mechanical and structural properties.

While the matching of arterial PCO_2 is well-defined both in concept and practice, the concept of MAP is fraught with problems. First, the value obtained for MAP depends on just where in the tracheobronchial tree the sampling catheter is placed, and for any such location, the orientation of the sampling port in the airway is also of importance. However, a still more fundamental issue is the rationale behind the use of MAP. Since HFV for general ventilatory support is directed towards the intensive care setting and the respiratory distress syndrome in which a cardinal feature is alveolar exudate, flooding, or atelectasis, the notion of the degree of lung expansion is critically important, just as it is with CMV and the use of PEEP. It seems that during HFV, MAP is sometimes taken to reflect mean alveolar pressure and hence the degree of lung expansion. While during CMV, mean airway and alveolar pressures may not be that different in the setting of alveolar filling (compared to the situation of airways obstruction) due to the low frequencies of breathing, such is clearly not the case for HFV. There is now considerable evidence that during HFV, mean alveolar pressure may considerably exceed MAP. This evidence comes from direct comparisons of alveolar and airway pressure by the alveolar capsule technique,[41] measurement of pressures along the airways,[42] and also indirectly from measurement of lung volume, showing a higher lung volume during HFV than CMV at the same MAP.[43,44] There appear to be several factors that can contribute to the difference between mean airway and alveolar pressures. Pressure measured in the large airways may be lower due to the Bernouilli effect; Fredberg[41] has suggested a pressure amplification phenomenon whereby alveolar pressures can exceed airway pressures, greatest at the resonant frequency; Simon et al.[45] has suggested that at least with some forms of HFV, the expiratory phase of each cycle may result in airway closure and thus, serve to reduce proximal airway pressure compared to alveolar. Since, as will be discussed, the major beneficial effect of HFV on gas exchange in some situations appears to be related to its ability to expand collapsed or fluid-filled alveoli, the concept and validity of matching MAP as a basis for comparing HFV and CMV should be carefully questioned at the time of experimental design in light of these arguments and observations.

With these issues in mind, comparisons of efficacy of CMV and HFV can now be addressed. Such studies have been done in species ranging from the rat to man, and a reasonable way to organize the information is by species.

Harf and colleagues[46] compared CMV to two combinations of CMV and HFOV that maintained the same tidal volume as with CMV alone in normal anesthetized rats. They found that the alveolar-arterial PO_2 difference ($AaDO_2$), which was 20 to 25 torr on CMV alone, fell by about 5 torr with both regimes of CMV plus HFOV. They felt this was best explained by improved $\dot{V}_A/\dot{Q}$ relationships due to better intrapulmonary gas mixing, and discounted increases in both effective ventilation and in cardiac output, or its distribution. While their conclusions may be correct, no hemodynamic measurements were made, and in particular, the effect of CMV plus HFOV on lung volume was not evaluated. A perfectly reasonable hypothesis (in line with the opening comment of this section) is that the large $AaDO_2$ (>20 torr) in normal rats during CMV alone was due to atelectasis, and that the addition of HFOV increased lung volume (PEEP-like effect), expanding atelectatic lung units and thus, improving gas exchange by a mechanism having nothing to do with gas mixing. Repeating this study with the animals breathing 100% O_2 would have permitted a clearer resolution of these competing hypotheses since, under these conditions, shunting and not $\dot{V}_A/\dot{Q}$ mismatch determines the $AaDO_2$: the $AaDO_2$ should fall with HFOV if re-expansion is the mechanism and should not change if improved gas mixing is the important issue. Measurement of lung volume on CMV and CMV plus HFOV would also have been helpful, but as it stands, whether HFOV per se is of benefit cannot be clearly inferred from the results.

The work of Kolton and co-workers[43] in the lung-injured rabbit strongly supports the importance of lung volume as the critical variable in the ventilatory strategy of HFV in pathologies characterized by edema, alveolar filling or atelectasis. Using both oleic acid-induced edema and surfactant depletion by lung lavage, these investigators showed considerably better oxygenation during HFOV than during CMV when MAP were equal and above critical airway opening pressures (mean PaO_2, 228 torr on HFOV vs. 71 torr on CMV). At the same time, lung volume was found to be higher during HFOV (58 mℓ above FRC) than during CMV (29 mℓ above FRC). Conversely, at MAP values below critical opening pressures, oxygenation and lung volumes were both low, and not different for the two forms of ventilation. Figure 2 shows the relationship between lung volume and arterial PO_2 constructed from all available average data in Kolton's paper (both CMV and HFOV data are shown for both disease models). It strongly supports the importance of lung volume, rather than the cause of the pulmonary lesion, MAP, or form of ventilation, as the important variable. The data strongly suggest that oxygenation is a function of lung volume rather than of the type of ventilation per se.

Kolton and co-workers, however, go on to point out consequences of the "equal volume — equal gas exchange" concept. At least in their hands, the level of PEEP required to reach volumes during CMV equal to those volumes during HFOV caused fatal pneumothorax on two occasions. Moreover, some lung units appeared to close at end-expiration during CMV with PEEP, while this did not happen with HFOV. As a result, the authors felt that in their experimental setting, adequate lung volumes and hence adequate gas exchange were more readily achieved with HFOV than CMV, with fewer complications. The authors, however, only fleetingly addressed the other important deleterious consequence of lung volume recruitment, namely, that of cardiovascular depression. They do briefly acknowledge loss of blood pressure during HFOV but state that it was reversible by administration of fluids. Hamilton et al.,[47] from the same group as Kolton, pursued the effect of HFOV in the lung-lavaged rabbit and extended the observations to include pathological examination. Again, HFOV mark-

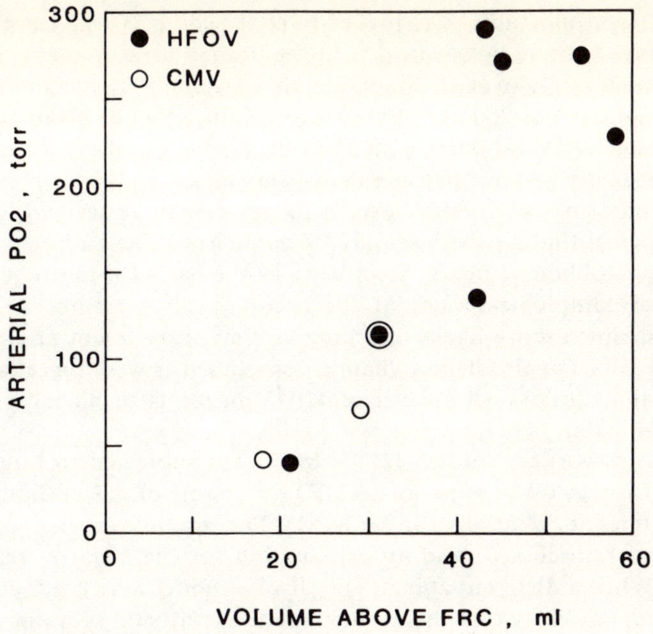

FIGURE 2. Relationship between arterial PO_2 and lung volume in rabbits with either oleic acid-induced pulmonary edema, or lung lavaged-induced surfactant deficiency. Data are from the paper by Kolton et al.[43] Solid circles refer to measurements made during HFOV, and open circles to measurements made during CMV. Each point is the mean of several animals. Note that arterial oxygenation is closely related to lung volume, and in particular, whether CMV or HFOV is used, and whether one considers oleic acid or lung lavage models appears to be of little importance. These data strongly support the notion that arterial oxygenation during HFV in models of alveolar filling or atelectasis depend more strongly on lung volume recruitment, rather than on the type of ventilation.

edly improved oxygenation and reduced pathological changes compared to CMV, but the protocol used matching of mean airway pressures at 15 cm H_2O for the two forms of ventilation, and unfortunately, measurements of lung volume were omitted. One wonders how the comparison may have turned out at matched lung volumes.

At this point, it is worth pointing out two important concepts in the analysis of these studies that must be considered prior to generalizing one's conclusions about the primary role of lung volume in maintenance of gas exchange. First, with these (and most) studies being carried out on 100% O_2, arterial PO_2 data reflect only the size of any shunt caused by atelectasis or alveolar filling, and permit absolutely no conclusions about how HFV may affect gas exchange in open, ventilated alveoli. Second, the disease models examined in these (and most) studies, namely, oleic acid-induced pulmonary edema and saline lavage-induced surfactant deficiency, are primarily models of atelectasis and alveolar filling in variable combination, resulting mainly in shunt rather than in $\dot{V}_A/\dot{Q}$ mismatch. Consequently, one must not necessarily expect similar results from HFV in diseases characterized by airways obstruction but without collapse or alveolar filling. More will be said about this issue later.

Other studies have been published comparing HFV and CMV in lung lavaged rabbits. Papers by Mook et al.[48] and Quan et al.[49] describe such comparisons. The work by Mook used both HFOV and HFVJ, but no lung volume measurements were made, nor hemodynamic indices recorded. MAP were different between HFOV (10 cm) and

HFJV (>10 cm) and mortality was higher with the latter. Clear-cut conclusions are almost impossible to draw, however, due to the limited measurements made and data reported. The paper of Quan et al. concluded that arterial PO_2 was significantly higher during HFJV than CMV (>200 vs. <100 torr respectively) while mean airway pressures were lower during HFJV (about 10 cm H_2O on HFVJ vs. about 15 cm H_2O during CMV). Again, no lung volume measurements were made, so the basis of the improved gas exchange cannot be determined, except to say that there seemed to be no differences in pathological findings between HFJV and CMV. The authors postulate either an increased lung volume or better gas mixing as the basis for improved PaO_2 during HFV. Given the pathologic nature of the lesion (hyaline membranes and alveolar edema), it seems much more likely that lung volume recruitment and not gas mixing was responsible. Once again, hemodynamic consequences were regrettably not evaluated either, so that the overall benefit of HFJV in terms of all important variables remains indeterminate.

Mammel and co-workers studied HFJV in the cat subjected to human meconium aspiration[50] and found CMV superior to HFJV in terms of gas exchange and pulmonary hemodynamics at essentially similar MAP. These results are in conflict with all of the preceding work discussed, and an explanation for the negative results would be worth finding. While a different animal and disease model were used, compared to the other studies, it is not likely that this would result in conflicting findings. One suspects differences in the application of HFVJ by the various investigators, but this is purely speculative, since the papers contain insufficient details for such an analysis. Again, the absence of lung volume measurement is seen to be a critical omission that impedes reaching clear-cut conclusions. Perhaps a clue in this particular paper is the relatively low mean airway pressures (less than 5 cm H_2O) prior to aspiration, with rather low values of end-expiratory pressure (2 cm H_2O) afterwards. It may well be that volume expansion of the lung was insufficient to overcome critical opening pressures, as so clearly described in Kolton's work.[43] Repeating the study, incorporating lung volume measurement and possibly adding sequences at higher mean pressures (and hence volumes) would potentially answer such questions, and might lead to different conclusions from those given.

Most comparisons of HFV and CMV have been carried out in dogs. In the normal dog, Chiaranda and co-workers[51] found arterial PO_2 to be similar when CMV was compared with HFJV at the same arterial PCO_2 and level of PEEP. The issue of lung volume also surfaces in this study because cardiovascular effects of the two modalities differed, possibly as a consequence of different lung volumes, which unfortunately were not measured. McEvoy et al.[52] compared gas exchange during CMV and HFOV in normal dogs and found that at similar mean airway pressures, arterial and mixed venous PO_2 and PCO_2 were similar for both forms of ventilation. So, too, were cardiac output and mean pulmonary artery pressure. This work was done before the importance of the lung volume-airway pressure relationship during HFV was generally appreciated, and so no lung volume measurements were made. These authors also examined steady state elimination of a mixture of inert gases of widely differing solubilities and molecular weight, and found no dependence of steady state elimination on molecular weight, an issue that will be addressed later in this chapter.

In contrast, the behavior of the very soluble gas acetone was found to be reproducibly very different from all gases of much lower solubility. Its elimination was found to be enhanced, an observation subsequently confirmed by Robertson and co-workers.[53] While this pattern of high acetone elimination is consistent with the development of lung units having high ventilation/perfusion ratio, no such units were found on direct analysis of the perfusion distribution by radioactive microsphere techniques.[52] It was subsequently shown that the probable mechanism for enhanced soluble gas elimination was facilitated transport of such gases in the liquid coating of the larger airways.[52] The respiratory gases are insufficiently soluble for this kind of facilitated transport to be of significance.

In McEvoy's study there was no evidence of abnormal exchange of poorly soluble gases, suggesting that HFOV was effective in maintaining ventilation to all lung regions and that it did not give rise to areas of low $\dot{V}_A/\dot{Q}$.

Thus, the papers of Chiaranda et al.[51] and of McEvoy et al.[52] using, respectively, HFJV and HFOV in normal dogs, both concluded that those modalities provided similar gas exchange at broadly similar airway pressures and levels of cardiovascular function, compared to CMV.

Oleic acid-induced pulmonary edema has been a popular model of respiratory distress in the dog for many years prior to the recent surge of interest in HFV. Recently, three studies have compared HFV and CMV in this model. While it is an interesting model, oleic acid-induced edema in the dog differs in important ways from clinical respiratory distress syndromes in man: the chest wall of the dog is much more compliant than that of man and makes ventilatory support by techniques aimed at recruiting lung volume (e.g., PEEP) generally more effective than in human disease. Moreover, the model produces severe pulmonary endothelial disruption, resulting in bloody fluid filling alveoli (a pathology quite different from that of exudates), inflammatory cells, hyaline membranes, and later fibrosis in human disease. The functional picture is that of fluid-filled alveoli, causing a shunt. Unaffected regions appear to function normally and areas of low $\dot{V}_A/\dot{Q}$ are generally absent. These differences are critical in attempting to reach conclusions concerning HFV in human respiratory distress syndromes from such dog studies and cannot be overemphasized.

In such an oleic acid model, Thompson and co-workers[54] found that HFOV and CMV at the same MAP were equivalent in terms of gas exchange and cardiovascular function. They concluded that: " . . . The mean airway pressure and presumably the mean lung volume, was of overwhelming importance" in accounting for this equivalence. Again, as with so many of the earlier studies of HFV, lung volume was not measured to clearly define its importance in gas exchange and cardiovascular function. There did not appear to be any difference in barotrauma incidence comparing HFV and CMV in this study. The clear-cut conclusion of the work is that cardiopulmonary function in canine oleic acid-induced edema depends mostly on lung volume, and whether adequate lung volumes are secured by CMV or HFOV is of little importance.

Schuster et al.[55] performed essentially similar studies, but compared CMV and HFJV (rather than HFOV) in the same dog model. Their results highlight the complexity of such comparative studies when "matching" of the two types of ventilation is done by indexes of airway pressure. They found HFJV inferior to CMV (for gas exchange) when: (1) PEEP level was the same for each mode; or (2) MAP was the same for each mode, but found HFJV superior to CMV for gas exchange at the same peak airway pressure, a situation resulting in a higher MAP during HFJV than during CMV. Once again, the absence of measurement of lung volume is lamented, and such absence prevents a clearer resolution of the comparability of the two forms of ventilation. However, the ventilatory modality better for gas exchange under any of these circumstances was associated with a lower cardiac output, and this does, in fact, suggest a lung volume-related effect on both. It seems entirely possible that if lung volumes had been matched, rather than one or other component of airway pressures, gas exchange and cardiovascular function may both have been similar for the two forms of ventilation.

Breen et al.[56] studied lobar oleic acid-induced edema in the dog and matched mean alveolar, rather than airway pressures, thus probably matching lung volumes. They found gas exchange equivalence and cardiovascular similarity under such conditions.

Lobar venous admixture was found to be sensitive to mean alveolar pressure, and "no intrinsic effect" of HFOV was demonstrable. Thus, these authors also conclude that lung volume recruitment is the basis for adequate gas exchange in this disease model, and that whether this is obtained via HFOV or CMV is not of importance. They do suggest that the smaller pressure oscillations of HFOV may protect against barotrauma at the same mean lung volume, but this is currently speculative.

Recently, two studies[57,58] have compared HFJV and CMV in surfactant depletion models in the dog, and once again, both conclude that under probably similar mechanical conditions, gas exchange is equivalent in terms of arterial PO_2 and PCO_2. However, as with almost all experiments reported, lung volume measurements were not made, and it is, thus, difficult to be sure how lung inflation compared between HFJV and CMV. Both groups felt that expansion of fluid-filled or collapsed alveoli was essential for restoration of gas exchange. In addition, Jibelian and Lachmann[58] summarize preliminary measurements made with the multiple inert gas elimination technique[59,60] in their surfactant-depleted dogs. They found that CMV with PEEP produced areas of high $\dot{V}_A/\dot{Q}$ just as noted by Dueck et al.[61] some years earlier, but during HFJV, inert gas elimination patterns suggested a much improved distribution of $\dot{V}_A/\dot{Q}$ ratios. Since the high $\dot{V}_A/\dot{Q}$ areas during CMV with PEEP have been shown to reflect decreased local perfusion as a consequence of over-distension,[62] they may be a good signal of impending barotrauma. Consequently, these findings, if substantiated by a formal study and report, suggest that HFJV in this circumstance may be advantageous under conditions of equivalent overall gas exchange compared to CMV.

HFOV has been compared to CMV in a premature primate model of infant respiratory distress.[63] HFOV produced a lower arterial PCO_2 than CMV, while arterial PO_2 was not different for the two regimes. At the same time, peak inspiratory pressure was higher during CMV, but there was no report of barotrauma with either mode, and postmortem studies of mechanical properties and lavaged phospholipids did not reveal any differences between HFOV and CMV. Neither lung volumes nor cardiovascular variables were measured, so a complete comparative profile of the two ventilatory modes cannot be made. While this report covered short term ventilation over the first few hours of life, a subsequent report from these authors[64] addresses the results of HFOV in the same model for a period of 24 hr, but again, without hemodynamic measurement or estimates of FRC. In this study, the results were the same as for the shorter term experiment. Arterial PO_2 was similar and arterial PCO_2 lower during HFOV compared to CMV. While MAP were not different, peak inspiratory pressures were high on CMV. No differences in total lung capacity, lavage phospholipids, wet/dry weight ratios or barotrauma were noted. A similar long term study of premature primates was undertaken by Bell and co-workers,[65] who extended the comparison of HFOV and CMV to about 96 hr of life. It is unfortunate that in this study, too, measurements of cardiac output, vascular pressures, and lung volumes were not reported, preventing a thorough comparison of the effect of the two ventilatory modes. The authors reach a conclusion strongly supportive of the pivotal role of lung volume in maintenance of gas exchange in respiratory distress models, as has been stressed above: it is probable that gas exchange equivalence depends on equivalent lung volumes in their study. There did not appear to be systematic pathological differences among the experimental groups which had been ventilated at similar, but not identical, MAP.

A few studies comparing HFV and CMV have been performed in man. Using HFPPV in 12 patients with adult respiratory distress syndromes of varying etiology, Wattwil et al.[66] found gas exchange, cardiovascular function, and patient acceptance similar to those under CMV at the same MAP. Schuster and co-workers[67] used HFJV in similar patients and reached identical conclusions: similar gas exchange and cardiac output at about the same MAP. They also found, as did Truog et al.[63] using HFOV, that peak inspiratory pressures were about 50% higher during CMV than during HFV at the same MAP, leading to speculations that HFV would reduce the incidence of barotrauma. However, as noted by Schuster, this potential advantage remains to be documented, both in animal models and man. In a subsequent paper from this group, Sladen et al.[68] compared HFJV and CMV in adults with acute respiratory failure using MAP of only about 5 cm H_2O (compared to about 17 cm H_2O in Schuster's work). Under these conditions, arterial PO_2 was substantially lower on HFJV (reminiscent of Mammel's work[50] at similar low MAP, as discussed earlier), while cardiac output was not different from that on CMV. Like virtually all studies, lung volume measurements were not made, but one would strongly suspect that at these lower airway pressures, HFJV was not maintaining alveoli open. Carlon and co-workers[69] performed a massive study using HFJV in 309 patients who needed ventilator support in the ICU. Their conclusions are strikingly similar to the above. HFJV and CMV produced similar results with respect to most variables including:

1. Survival
2. Duration of stay in the ICU
3. Incidence of barotrauma
4. Cardiac output
5. Gas exchange

The paper does not report MAP, and lung volumes were not measured.

Hurst and DeHaven[70] compared CMV (in the form of intermittent mandatory ventilation plus continuous positive airway pressure; IMV/CPAP) with HFJV in combination with zero, one or two IMV breaths/min in 9 patients with respiratory failure. Very few data are presented, and in particular, only arterial PO_2 and PCO_2 are depicted. Without knowing effects on MAP and lung volumes, the most general interpretation of the results of their paper is that, as with the preceding studies, HFJV was of little or no advantage compared to CMV. No data are given with respect to potential complications.

Finally, Rouby et al. used HFJV in 24 patients with respiratory failure.[71] These authors found a very close correlation between MAP and arterial PO_2 as shown in Figure 3, reproduced from their paper. Moreover, an equally good relationship exists between lung volume and arterial PO_2 (Figure 4), using mean data obtained from their paper. Thus, these results are compatible with the data of Kolton et al.[43] in Figure 2, and support the general conclusions culled from all studies reviewed to this point. It is unfortunate that the only indexes of cardiovascular function monitored were arterial pressure and heart rate. It would have been very useful to know about how lung volume recruitment affected cardiac output, since increases in FRC by almost 2 ℓ were achieved during HFJV at MAP in excess of 30 cm H_2O. While no report of barotrauma is given in Rouby's paper, one must be concerned using HFJV at such high mean pressures, in terms of both lung damage and cardiovascular depression.

A. Summary of Studies Comparing CMV and HFV

All of the comparative studies described above come to remarkably similar conclusions. This is all the more surprising because the several studies encompass:

1. Many different laboratories
2. Many different techniques of HFV
3. Many different species, from rat to man
4. Variations in pathology from none to life-threatening alveolar filling, flooding and/or atelectasis from respiratory distress syndromes
5. Ages fron newborn to the 8th decade

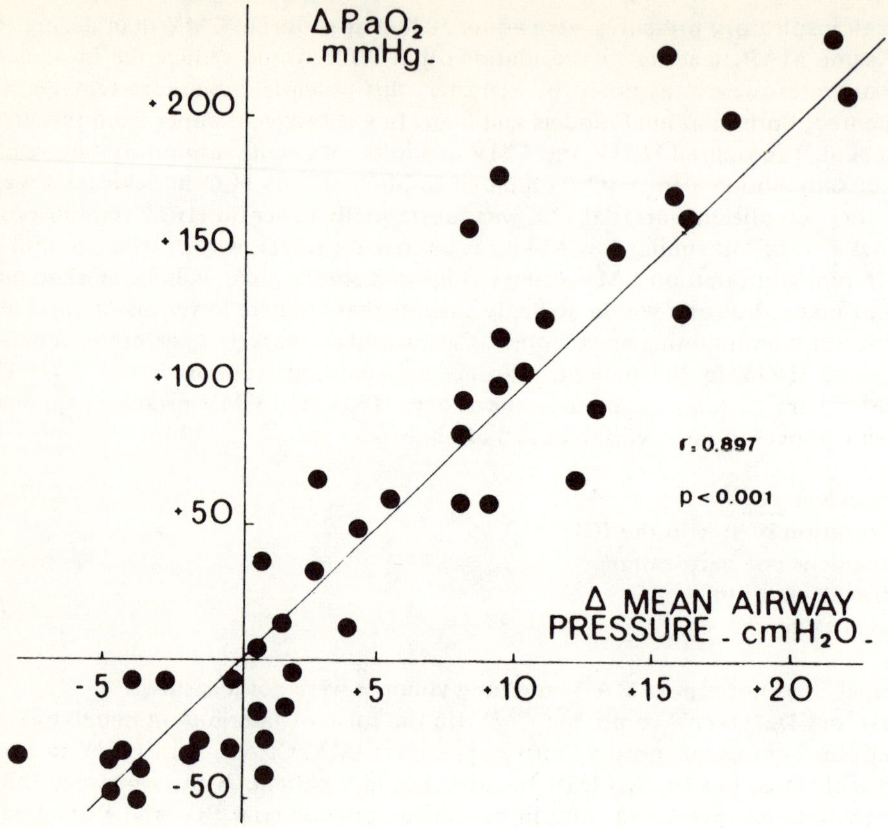

FIGURE 3. Relationship between the change in arterial PO_2 and change in MAP during HFJV in 15 patients with respiratory distress. Data are from Rouby et al.[71] The origin of the axes refers to intermittent positive pressure ventilation conditions. In this particular study, mean airway and alveolar pressures were identical, and thus it is reasonable to infer that the abscissa of this figure is also representative of lung volume. There is a clear-cut relationship between arterial oxygenation and this index of lung expansion. Note that while Figure 2 refers to rabbits with induced lung disease and HFOV, the data in this figure are for post-operative patients studied with HFJV. (From Rouby, J. J. et al., Anesthesiology, 59, 281, 1983. With permission.)

Stripped of fine points, the major, overwhelming conclusion is that HFV and CMV produce equivalent arterial oxygenation at equivalent lung volumes and arterial PCO_2 levels. Furthermore, under such equivalent conditions:

1. Cardiovascular function appears essentially similar, at least in terms of cardiac ouput.
2. No evidence has been produced that HFV reduces the risk of barotrauma compared to CMV. The latter conclusion is reached in spite of general agreement that *peak* inspiratory pressures are as much as 50% higher on CMV than HFV, even when MAP are the same.
3. No evidence of lung damage or altered surfactant metabolism has been found as long as humidified gas is inspired and care is taken with the physical arrangement of the jet in HFJV.

Minor deviations from these conclusions probably reflect minor differences in either HFV hardware or techniques of application.

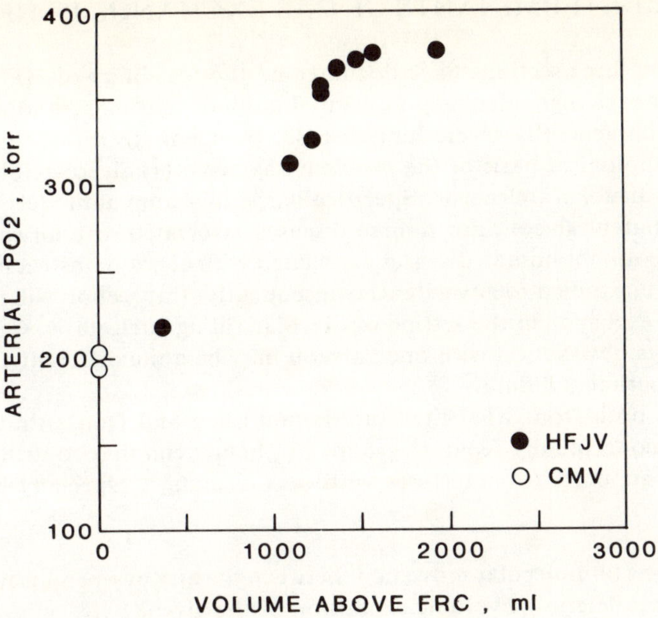

FIGURE 4. Further data from the paper by Rouby et al., as in Figure 3, showing arterial PO_2 as a function of volume above FRC for a total of 24 patients ventilated by HFJV post-operatively. Each point represents the mean of at least 9 patients, and closed circles refer to different ways of applying HFJV, namely, by varying either I/E ratio or frequency. There is a clear-cut relationship between arterial PO_2 and lung volume, independently of the way in which HFV is applied.

However, in coming to these conclusions, it seems critical to keep in mind the nature of the pulmonary pathology being treated with HFV. In the acute animal models and the neonatal and adult respiratory distress syndromes studied to date, the pathological process is dominated by focal alveolar filling, flooding, or atelectasis. It seems entirely logical then, that for such a process, the key to successful gas exchange is adequate alveolar expansion. It would not seem important how such expansion is achieved, and it further seems reasonable that cardiac output reduction will reflect such lung volume changes rather than the mode of ventilation, as has been found to be the case so far.

Conversely, in lung diseases characterized not by alveolar pathology, but by airways obstruction proximal to patent, normal alveoli, the efficacy of HFV may be altogether different. Such diseases or their animal model counterparts are very difficult to study, both because no adequate stable animal model exists, and because to properly study such a model and its responses to HFV requires methods of directly measuring $\dot{V}_A/\dot{Q}$ inequality (rather than the more readily measured shunt fractions that are more important in respiratory distress syndromes).

Finally, for useful comparisons of HFV and CMV, it appears important to make simultaneous measurements of gas exchange, airway pressures, cardiovascular pressures and flows, and most importantly, *lung volume.* With two notable exceptions (the papers of Kolton et al.[43] and Rouby et al.[71]), lung volume measurements are lacking. Because of the previously noted difficulties in measuring MAP and relating them to lung volume in CMV and HFV, the lack of volume measurements seriously interferes with one's ability to reach clear-cut conclusions concerning the efficacy of HFV.

V. DETERMINANTS OF GAS EXCHANGE IN HFV

The preceding three sections have documented the feasibility of HFV (of all types) in terms of gas exchange adequacy in normal animals and man, and also in animals and patients with generally severe lung disease. In essentially all of the diseased lung studies, the pathological basis of the problem has been: (1) alveolar filling by fluid or exudate; or (2) alveolar atelectasis. Specifically, neither animal models of airways obstruction with patent alveoli, nor human diseases associated with airways obstruction with patent alveoli, nor human diseases associated with airways obstruction but normal alveoli, have been studied to any extent. Consequently, this section will focus on determinants of gas exchange in the setting of alveolar filling/atelectasis. Conclusions pertinent to airways obstruction with open alveoli may be quite different and must await appropriate experimental data.

It is evident, both from what literature is published and from intuitive logic, that there are *three* conceptually separate groups of phenomena that contribute to the way in which HFV supports (or interferes with) gas exchange, especially in the alveolar filling diseases:

1. Mechanisms of molecular movement between the airway opening and the alveoli.
2. Factors that determine volume expansion of the alveoli.
3. Potential effects of HFV on distribution of bloodflow.

A. Molecular Movement between the Airway Opening and Alveoli

There is abundant evidence that several physical transport phenomena co-exist and must contribute to the movement of molecules up and down the tracheobronchial tree in HFV. In spite of much theoretical and experimental work, uncertainty still exists as to what extent these several mechanisms are each responsible for transport under any particular set of conditions. Only a short personal viewpoint will be given here because this enormously complex subject is better and more extensively treated elsewhere.

It is generally agreed, as stated by Slutsky,[72] that there can be only two physical processes involved, namely, convection and diffusion. The relative importance of each, and particularly any interaction between the two, may be different during HFV as compared to CMV. In a different vein, the high velocity of gas flow produced by HFV implies that regional distribution of gas molecules will depend rather differently on the basic mechanical factors so long considered in CMV. It is generally held that compliance of lung tissue is not as important at high frequencies, while resistance retains a major role. However, inertial factors not important in CMV must play an increasingly important role in determining flow patterns when frequency is increased. One experimentally observed consequence of this rearrangement of the importance of mechanical factors is that of apparent circulating currents.[73] By means of stroboscopic photography, it was shown that regional lung movements were considerably out of phase with one another, and subsequent radioactive gas measurements suggest that this phenomenon results in rapid gas mixing *between* large regions in the normal lung.[74] However, since most of the significant impediments to gas exchange in disease relate to abnormalities in ventilation or bloodflow at a much finer level of spatial resolution, the biological significance of these findings is not at all clear. Data reviewed in this chapter, in fact suggest no identifiable role for this phenomenon, since, at the same lung volume, CMV and HFV produce equivalent oxygenation. A caveat to this conclusion is the very preliminary data of Jibelian and Lachmann[58] who may have observed less $\dot{V}_A/\dot{Q}$ inequality during HFV than during CMV in a surfactant deficient model.

Another major proposed effect of HFV in terms of gas transport is the potentially increased interaction between diffusion and convection suggested by Fredberg.[75] While this theory was developed independently of Lehr's circulating currents concept, Lehr's mechanism might be subject to the same interaction proposed by Fredberg for more direct inspiratory ventilation. In relation to Fredberg's work, considerable evidence is now available to document the insensitivity of the transport of insoluble inert gases to molecular weight during HFV. Robertson et al.[53,76] found that resident gas density affected gas exchange during HFV in the same manner as during CMV. McEvoy et al.,[52] Knopp et al.,[77] and Kaethner et al.[78] all concluded that overall gas transport was negligibly, if at all, affected by molecular weight differences, using gases as different in molecular weight as He and SF_6 (MW of 4 and 146). It would seem unlikely that if enhanced interaction between convection and diffusion were critical, gas transport would be insensitive to molecular weight. Chakrabarti et al.[79] came to similar conclusions studying CO_2 elimination.

Another mechanism postulated is that even if total tidal volume is less than the average anatomic deadspace during HFV, alveoli more proximal than average may still be ventilated[80] in the conventional, convective sense. This certainly seems reasonable in view of the known anatomy. Other convective phenomena such as the asymmetry between inspiration and expiration produced by bronchial bifurcations[81] may be of importance in HFV, but this remains to be documented. Liquid model analogs of HFV permit hydrodynamically equivalent oscillations to be observed at much lower frequencies, allowing direct observation of flow profiles marked by dye. Such studies seem to show that in a branching airway network there is considerable mixing in large common airways, such that rapid interregional dispersion of dye marker is reproducibly seen.[82]

The similarity in gas exchange between CMV and HFV (at similar lung volumes) in disease models discussed earlier, and the evidence refuting diffusion limitation for insoluble inert gases, suggests that bulk flow mechanisms remain important and dominant in transporting molecules to/from the gas exchange region.

B. Factors that Determine Volume Expansion of the Alveoli

In alveolar filling/collapse situations, a thorough review of the literature as presented herein leaves one with the overwhelming sense of the importance of lung volume. In fact, when HFV and CMV are compared at similar lung volumes, they appear to generate equivalent gas exchange. Furthermore, there are excellent correlations between lung volume and arterial PO_2 that encompass different forms of ventilation (CMV and HFV), different operational parameters of ventilation, and different pathological processes in different species (Figures 2, 3, and 4).

It is, therefore, difficult to refute the pivotal role of lung volume recruitment in gas exchange maintenance. As previously agreed, such a role for lung volume is intuitively and logically reasonable in light of the pathology one is attempting to deal with.

It would seem that the most important questions that can now be posed for HFV relate to whether complications and long term outcome are any different when animals or patients are compared on the two ventilatory modes at similar lung volumes. In other words, the short term issue of comparative efficacy of CMV and HFV seems largely settled for the diseases related to alveolar filling or collapse: as long as the same lung volumes are reached, gas exchange is equivalent.

This rather simple conclusion should be tempered by the observations of the Toronto group with respect to critical airway opening pressures.[43] While CMV and HFV may be equivalent at any lung volume, they will only be adequate at volumes that prevent collapse of most of the alveoli at end-expiration.

The question of the role of lung volume recruitment in obstructive diseases with open alveoli will be far more difficult to answer since animal models of this are very unstable or transient, and also because there is less need for ventilatory support for such patients compared to the respiratory distress group addressed earlier. Intuitively, one would not expect that lung volume will become a critical issue. Rather, under such circumstances, the various factors discussed above which affect airway gas transport must become more important. The only experimental comparison of HFV and CMV in such a pathological state reported in fact, very similar conclusions to those during alveolar filling or collapse:[83] no benefit from HFV compared to CMV. However, more work should be done in models of airway obstruction before the role of HFV can be properly defined in such a setting.

C. Potential Effects of HFV on the Distribution of Bloodflow

In normal dogs, Brusasco et al.[74] found little or no difference between topographical distribution of perfusion during CMV and HFV, as had McEvoy et al. previously.[52] Moreover, McEvoy and co-workers[52] searched for, but did not find, any radial gradient in bloodflow that might have been postulated to occur on the basis of pressure dissipation along the airways during HFOV.

There has only been one study published to date that directly examines distribution of bloodflow to the lung in the presence of disease. Hall et al.[84] compared by flow probes the distribution of bloodflow between a collapsed left lung and expanded right lung during CMV and HFOV. They found that fractional perfusion of the collapsed lung was lower during HFOV than during CMV (32 vs. 37% of cardiac output). Venous admixture differences were similar, yet arterial PO_2 was much higher on HFOV. This finding is almost certainly due to the observation that cardiac output during HFOV was more than 50% greater than during CMV. In turn, this can be explained by the considerably lower intrapleural pressures (-6 cm with HFOV, -3 cm with CMV) which probably reflect different degrees of lung inflation. Presumably, if MAP had been raised during HFOV to provide equivalent lung volumes, cardiac output would have been lower, and the relative hyperinflation of the noncollapsed right lung may well have diverted bloodflow back to the collapsed left lung. Thus, at the same lung volumes, one might postulate no difference between CMV and HFOV with respect to distribution of perfusion. It would be most useful to carry out further studies of the type reported by Hall, including measurement of right lung volume, and to repeat measurements over a range of matched lung volumes during CMV and HFOV. Such experiments would considerably clarify the role of lung distension in affecting perfusion distribution, an area of obvious importance in HFV that has received essentially no attention. Kapitan et al.[85] reported observations consistent with these notions in a dog model of unilateral hypoventilation. At equal MAP, the nonobstructed lung was relatively hyperinflated during HFOV compared to CMV. This clearly diverted bloodflow from the well-ventilated to the poorly ventilated lung and adversely affected gas exchange. In this way, volume recruitment during HFV may produce similar results as are known to occur with CMV with PEEP: improvement by expanding and ventilating previously collapsed alveoli, but also potential decrements in gas exchange due to redistribution of perfusion away from well-ventilated units. Again, this kind of effect is almost certainly lung expansion-dependent and has little or nothing to do with mechanisms of molecular transport between the airway opening and the alveolar region.

VI. SUMMARY AND CONCLUSIONS

In summary, a host of airway transport mechanisms probably co-exist and account for adequate molecular movement between the airway opening and the alveolar region. Most evidence suggests that such movement is not diffusion-limited. The relative importance of the several possible convective mechanisms remains to be sorted out.

In diseases characterized by alveolar filling or atelectasis, the overwhelming factor that determines adequacy of gas exchange appears to be lung volume recruitment (and under such conditions, whether CMV or HFOV is used is relatively unimportant). This conclusion demands that lung volumes be measured in studies of HFV and be used as the basis for comparison to CMV, rather than the commonly used index of MAP which is both difficult to measure and hard to interpret.

How HFV affects pulmonary perfusion distribution is of major importance, and is only just beginning to be studied. Data obtained so far indicate that the principal determinant of how the perfusion distribution is modified by HFV is, as with CMV, related to how normal lung units are expanded by the ventilatory mode compared to fluid-filled or collapsed units. Potentially deleterious distribution away from well-ventilation alveoli may take place with overinflation.

HFV can certainly support adequate gas exchange for extended periods of time, even in critically ill patients. Whether HFV has any advantage in terms of complications such as barotrauma or cardiovascular depression remains to be determined, but at this time there is no convincing evidence of any advantage when comparisons to CMV are made at similar lung volumes, except in special situations such as thoracic surgery, air leak syndromes and other particular circumstances.

REFERENCES

1. Jonzon, A., Obert, P. A., Sedin, G., and Sjostrand, U., High-frequency positive-pressure ventilation by endotracheal insufflation, *Acta Anaesth. Scand.*, Suppl. 43, 4, 1971.
2. Jonzon, A., Sedin, G., and Sjostrand, U., High-frequency positive-pressure ventilation (HFPPV) applied for small lung ventilation and compared with spontaneous respiration and continuous positive airway pressure (CPAP), *Acta Anaesth. Scand.*, Suppl. 53, 23, 1973.
3. Fletcher, P. R. and Epstein, R. A., Constancy of physiological dead space during high-frequency ventilation, *Respir. Physiol.*, 47, 39, 1982.
4. Jonzon, A., Rondio, Z., and Sedin, G., Alveolar deadspace during high frequency positive pressure ventilation, *Br. J. Anaesth.*, 55, 1133, 1983.
5. Pinchak, A. C., Hagen, J. F., Hancock, D., and Kovijanic, C., High-frequency positive-pressure ventilation with the MA-1 ventilator, *Crit. Care Med.*, 12(9), 810, 1984.
6. Klain, M. and Smith, R. B., High frequency percutaneous transtracheal jet ventilation, *Crit. Care Med.*, 5(6), 280, 1977.
7. Smith, R. B., Cutaia, F., Hoff, B. H., Babinski, M., and Gelineau, J., Long-term transtracheal high frequency ventilation in dogs, *Crit. Care Med.*, 9(4), 311, 1981.
8. Mihm, F. G., Feeley, T. W., and Rodarte, A., Monitoring end-tidal carbon dioxide tensions with high-frequency jet ventilation in dogs with normal lungs, *Crit. Care Med.*, 12(3), 180, 1984.
9. Lunkenheimer, P. P., Rafflenbeul, P., Keller, H., Frank, I., Dickhut, H. H., and Fuhrmann, C., *Br. J. Anesth.*, 44, 627, 1972.
10. Bohn, D. J., Miyasaka, K., Marchak, B. E., Thompson, W. K., Froese, A. B., and Bryan, A. C., Ventilation by high-frequency oscillation, *J. Appl. Physiol.*, 48(4), 710, 1980.
11. Butler, W. J., Bohn, D. J., Bryan, A. C., and Froese, A. B., Ventilation by high-frequency oscillation in humans, *Anesth. Analg.*, 59, 577, 1980.
12. Rieke, H., Hook, C., and Meyer, M., Pulmonary gas exchange during high-frequency ventilation in dogs, *Respir. Physiol.*, 54, 1, 1983.
13. Rehder, K., Schmid, E. R., and Knopp, T. J., Long-term high-frequency ventilation in dogs, *Am. Rev. Respir. Dis.*, 128, 476, 1983.
14. Bitterman, H., Kerem, D. H., Shabati, Y., Gavriely, N., and Palti, Y., Respiration maintained by externally applied vibration and tracheal insufflation in the cat, *Anesth. Analg.*, 62, 33, 1983.
15. Zidulka, A., Gross, D., Minami, H., Vartian, V., and Chang, H. K., Ventilation by high-frequency chest wall compression in dogs with normal lungs, *Am. Rev. Respir. Dis.*, 127, 709, 1983.
16. Harf, A., Bertrand, C., and Chang, H. K., Ventilation by high-frequency oscillation of thorax or at trachea in rats, *J. Appl. Physiol.*, 56(1), 155, 1984.

17. Doyle, H. J., Napolitano, A. E., Lippman, H. R., Cooper, K. R., Duncan, J. S., Eakins, K., and Glauser, F. L., Different humidification systems for high-frequency jet ventilation, *Crit. Care Med.*, 12(9), 815, 1984.
18. Ramanathan, S., Sinha, K., Arismendy, J., Chalon, J., and Turndorf, H., Humidification and airway pressures during high-frequency jet ventilation delivered through the suction-biopsy channel of a flexible bronchofiberscope, *Crit. Care Med.*, 12(9), 820, 1984.
19. Frank, I., Noack, W., Lunkenheimer, P. P., Ising, H., Keller, H., Dickhuth, H. H., Rafflenbeul, W., and Jacobson, M., Light- and electron microscopic investigations of pulmonary tissue after high-frequency positive-pressure ventilation (HFPPV), *Anesthesiology*, 171, 1975.
20. Frantz, I. D., III, Stark, A. R., Davis, J. M., Davies, P., and Kitzmiller, T. J., High-frequency ventilation does not affect pulmonary surfactant, liquid, or morphologic features in normal cats, *Am. Rev. Respir. Dis.*, 26, 909, 982.
21. Keszler, M., Klein, R., McClellan, L., Nelson, D., and Platt, M., Effects of conventional and high frequency jet ventilation on lung parenchyma, *Crit. Care Med.*, 10(8), 514, 1982.
22. Ophoven, J. P., Mammel, M. C., Gordon, M. J., and Boros, S. J., Tracheobronchial histopathology associated with high-frequency jet ventilation, *Crit. Care Med.*, 12(9), 829, 1984.
23. Bland, R. D., Kim, M. H., Light, M. J., and Woodson, J. L., High frequency mechanical ventilation in severe hyaline membrane disease. An alternative treatment?, *Crit. Care Med.*, 8(5), 275, 1980.
24. Frantz, I. D., III, Werthammer, J., and Stark, A. R., High-frequency ventilation in premature infants with lung disease: adequate gas exchange at low tracheal pressure, *Pediatrics*, 71(4), 483, 1983.
25. Barzilay, E., Lev, A., Lesmes, C., Fleck, R., and Khourieh, A., Combined use of HFPPV with low-rate ventilation in traumatic respiratory insufficiency, *Intensive Care Med.*, 10, 197, 1984.
26. Eyal, F. G., Arad, I. D., Godder, K., and Robinson, M. J., High-frequency positive-pressure ventilation in neonates, *Crit. Care. Med.*, 12(9), 793, 1984.
27. Scheck, P. A. and Mallios, C., Peroral endoscopies using intravenous anesthesia and high-frequency ventilation, *Crit. Care Med.*, 12(9), 803, 1984.
28. Schuster, D. P., Snyder, J. V., Klain, M., and Grenvik, A., High-frequency jet ventilation during the treatment of acute fulminant pulmonary edema, *Chest*, 80(6), 682, 1981.
29. Ashley, M., Cameron, A. E., and Slee, I. P., High frequency jet ventilation — Its use in respiratory insufficiency, *Intensive Care Med.*, 8, 257, 1983.
30. Sladen, A., Guntupalli, K., Marquez, J., and Klain, M., High-frequency jet ventilation in the postoperative period: a review of 100 patients, *Crit. Care Med.*, 12(9), 782, 1984.
31. Seki, S., Goto, K., Kondo, T., Fukushima, Y., Konishi, H., and Kosaka, F., Gas exchange and facilitation of high-frequency ventilation in intrathoracic surgery, *Ann. Thorac. Surg.*, 37(6), 491, 1984.
32. Mutz, N., Baum, M., Benzer, H., Koller, W., Moritz, E., and Pauser, G., Intraoperative application of high-frequency ventilation, *Crit. Care Med.*, 12(9), 800, 1984.
33. Klain, M., Kalla, R., Sladen, A., and Guntupalli, K., High-frequency jet ventilation in weaning the ventilator-dependent patient, *Crit. Care Med.*, 12(9), 780, 1984.
34. Johnston, J. R., Coppel, D. L., Wilson, J. J., McLaughlin, B. F., and Hildebrand, P. J., High frequency jet ventilation, *Anaesthesia*, 39, 163, 1984.
35. Mendez, M., Pratt, D. S., and May, J. J., Prolonged high-frequency jet ventilation, *Crit. Care Med.*, 12(9), 838, 1984.
36. Neu, J., Hamilton, L., Linehan, J., Rich, M., Murkowski, K., Wilson, A., and Oechler, H., Long-term high-frequency jet ventilation in neonates, *Crit. Care Med.*, 12(9), 833, 1984.
37. Nishimura, M., Takezawa, J., Nishijima, M. K., Taenaka, N., Shimada, Y., Yoshiya, I., and Fujimoto, Y., High-frequency jet ventilation for differential lung ventilation, *Crit. Care Med.*, 12(9), 840, 1984.
38. Wright, K., Lyrene, R. K., Truog, W. E., Standaert, T. A., Murphy, J., and Woodrum, D. E., Ventilation by high-frequency oscillation in rabbits with oleic acid lung disease, *J. Appl. Physiol.*, 50(5), 1056, 1981.
39. Marchak, B. E., Thompson, W. K., Duffty, P., Miyaki, T., Bryan, M. H., Bryan, A. C., and Froese, A. B., Treatment of RDS by high-frequency oscillatory ventilation: a preliminary report, *Pediatrics*, 99(2), 287, 1981.
40. Boynton, B. R., Mannino, F. L., Davis, R. F., Kopotic, R. J., and Friederichsen, G., Combined high-frequency oscillatory ventilation and intermittent mandatory ventilation in critically ill neonates, *J. Pediatr.*, 105(2), 297, 1984.
41. Fredberg, J. J., Keefe, D. H., Glass, G. M., Castile, R. G., and Frantz, I. D., III, Alveolar pressure nonhomogenity during small-amplitude high-frequency oscillation, *J. Appl. Physiol.*, 57(3), 788, 1984.
42. Sutton, J. E. and Glass, D., Airway pressure gradient during high-frequency ventilation, *Crit. Care Med.*, 12(9), 774, 1984.

43. Kolton, M., Cattran, C. B., Kent, G., Volgysei, G., Froese, A. B., and Bryan, A. C., Oxygenation during high-frequency ventilation compared with conventional mechanical ventilation in two models of lung injury, *Anesth. Analg.*, 61(4), 323, 1982.
44. Saari, A. F., Rossing, T. H., Solway, J., and Drazen, J. M., Lung inflation during high-frequency ventilation, *Am. Rev. Respir. Dis.*, 129, 333, 1984.
45. Simon, B. A., Weinmann, G. G., and Mitzner, W., Mean airway pressure and alveolar pressure during high-frequency ventilation, *J. Appl. Physiol.*, 57(4), 1069, 1984.
46. Harf, A., Le Gall, R., and Chang, H. K., Mechanical ventilation with superimposed high frequency oscillation in the normal rat, *Respir. Physiol.*, 54, 31, 1983.
47. Hamilton, P. P., Onayemi, A., Smyth, J. A., Gillan, J. E., Cutz, E., Froese, A. B., and Bryan, A. C., Comparison of conventional and high-frequency ventilation: oxygenation and lung pathology, *J. Appl. Physiol.*, 55(1), 1983.
48. Mook, P. H., Proctor, H. J., Zee, H. V. D., Ennema, J. J., and Wildevuur, Ch. R. H., High-frequency ventilation in rabbits with respiratory insufficiency, *J. Surg. Res.*, 36, 614, 1984.
49. Quan, S. F., Militzer, H. W., Calkins, J. M., Sobonya, R. E., Waterson, C. K., Otto, C. W., and Conahan, T. J., Comparison of high-frequency jet ventilation with conventional mechanical ventilation in saline-lavaged rabbits, *Crit. Care Med.*, 12(9), 759, 1984.
50. Mammel, M. C., Gordon, M. J., Connett, J. E., and Boros, S. J., Comparison of high-frequency jet ventilation and conventional mechanical ventilation in a meconium aspiration model, *Pediatrics*, 103(4), 630, 1983.
51. Chiaranda, M., Rubini, A., Fiore, G., Giron, G., and Carion, G. C., Hemodynamic effects of continuous positive-pressure ventilation and high-frequency jet ventilation with positive end-expiratory pressure in normal dogs, *Crit. Care Med.*, 12(9), 750, 1984.
52. McEvoy, R. D., Davies, N. J. H., Mannino, F. L., Prutow, R. J., Schumacker, P. T., Wagner, P. D., and West, J. B., Pulmonary gas exchange during high-frequency ventilation, *J. Appl. Physiol.*, 52(5), 1278, 1982.
53. Robertson, H. T., Coffey, R. L., Standaert, T. A., and Truog, W. E., Respiratory and inert gas exchange during high-frequency ventilation, *J. Appl. Physiol.*, 52(3), 683, 1982.
54. Thompson, W. K., Marchak, B. E., Froese, A. B., and Bryan, A. C., High-frequency oscillation compared with standard ventilation in pulmonary injury model, *J. Appl. Physiol.*, 52(3), 543, 1982.
55. Schuster, D. P., Snyder, J. V., and Klain, M., Comparison of venous admixture during high-frequency ventilation and conventional ventilation in oleic acid-induced pulmonary edema in dogs, *Anesth. Analg.*, 61(9), 735, 1982.
56. Breen, P. H., Ali, J., and Wood, L. D. H., High-frequency ventilation in lung edema: effects on gas exchange and perfusion, *J. Appl. Physiol.*, 56(1), 187, 1984.
57. Kumar, B. S., Beney, K., Jastremski, M., Nieman, G., and Bredenberg, C., High-frequency jet ventilation versus conventional ventilation after surfactant displacement in dogs, *Crit. Care Med.*, 12(9), 738, 1984.
58. Jibelian, G. and Lachmann, B., Gas exchange during conventional and high-frequency pulse ventilation in the surfactant-deficient lung: influence of positive end-expiratory pressure, *Crit. Care Med.*, 12(9), 769, 1984.
59. Wagner, P. D., Naumann, P. F., and Laravuso, R. B., Simultaneous measurement of eight foreign gases in blood by gas chromatography, *J. Appl. Physiol.*, 36, 600, 1974.
60. Evans, J. W. and Wagner, P. D., Limits on $\dot{V}_A/\dot{Q}$ distributions from analysis of experimental inert gas elimination, *J. Appl. Physiol.*, 42, 889, 1977.
61. Dueck, R., Wagner, P. D., and West, J. B., Effects of PEEP on gas exchange in dogs with normal and edematous lungs, *Anesthesiology*, 47, 359, 1977.
62. Hedenstierna, G., White, F. C., Mazzone, R. W., and Wagner, P. D., Redistributions of pulmonary blood flow in the dog with PEEP ventilation, *J. Appl. Physiol.*, 46, 372, 1979.
63. Truog, W. E., Standaert, T. A., Murphy, J., Palmer, S., Woodrum, D. E., and Hodson, W. A., Effect of high-frequency oscillation on gas exchange and pulmonary phospholipids in experimental hyaline membrane disease, *Am. Rev. Respir. Dis.*, 127, 585, 1983.
64. Truog, W. E., Standaert, T. A., Murphy, J. H., Woodrum, D. E., and Hodson, W. A., Effects of prolonged high-frequency oscillatory ventilation in premature primates with experimental hyaline membrane disease, *Am. Rev. Respir. Dis.*, 130, 76, 1984.
65. Bell, R. E., Kuehl, T. J., Coalson, J. J., Ackerman, N. B., Null, D. M., Escobedo, M. B., Yoder, B. A., Cornish, J. D., Nalle, L., Skarin, R. M., Cipriani, C. A., Montes, M., Robotham, J. L., and DeLemos, R. A., High-frequency ventilation in the treatment of hyaline membrane disease in primates, *Crit. Care Med.*, 12(9), 764, 1984.
66. Wattwil, L. M., Sjostrand, U. H., and Borg, U. R., Comparative studies of IPPV and HFPPV with PEEP in critical care patients. I. A clinical evaluation, *Crit. Care Med.*, 11(1), 30, 1983.

67. Schuster, D. P., Klain, M., and Snyder, J. V., Comparison of high frequency jet ventilation to conventional during severe acute respiratory failure in humans, *Crit. Care Med.*, 10(10), 625, 1982.
68. Sladen, A., Guntupalli, K., and Klain, M., High-frequency versus intermittent positive-pressure ventilation, *Crit. Care Med.*, 12(9), 788, 1984.
69. Carlon, G. C., Howland, W. S., Ray, C., Miodownik, S., Griffin, J. P., and Groeger, J. S., High-frequency jet ventilation: a prospective randomized evaluation, *Chest*, 84, 551, 1983.
70. Hurst, J. M. and DeHaven, C. B., Adult respiratory distress syndrome: improved oxygenation during high-frequency jet ventilation/continuous positive airway pressure, *Surgery*, 96(4), 764, 1984.
71. Rouby, J. J., Fusciardi, J., Bourgain, J. L., and Viars, P., High-frequency jet ventilation in postoperative respiratory failure: determinants of oxygenation, *Anesthesiology*, 59, 281, 1983.
72. Slutsky, A., Mechanisms affecting gas transport during high-frequency oscillation, *Crit. Care Med.*, 12(9), 713, 1984.
73. Lehr, J. L., Butler, J. P., Westerman, P. A., Zantz, S. L., and Drazen, J. M., Photographic measurement of pleural surface motion during lung oscillation, *J. Appl. Physiol.*, in press, 1985.
74. Brusasco, V., Knopp, T. J., Schmid, E. R., and Rehder, K., Ventilation-perfusion relationship during high-frequency ventilation, *J. Appl. Physiol.*, 56(2), 454, 1984.
75. Fredberg, J. J., Augmented diffusion in the airways can support pulmonary gas exchange, *J. Appl. Physiol.*, 49(2), 232, 1980.
76. Robertson, H. T., Coffey, R. L., and Hlastala, M., Influence of carrier gas density on gas exchange during high frequency ventilation, *Bull. Eur. Physiopathol. Resp.*, 18, 381, 1982.
77. Knopp, T. J., Kaethner, T., Meyer, M., Rehder, K., and Scheid, P., Gas mixing in the airways of dog lungs during high-frequency ventilation, *J. Appl. Physiol.*, 55(4), 1141, 1983.
78. Kaethner, T., Kohl, J., and Scheid, P., Gas concentration profiles along airways of dog lungs during high-frequency ventilation, *J. Appl. Physiol.*, 56(6), 1491, 1984.
79. Chakrabarti, M. K., Loh, L., and Gilchrist, I., High frequency ventilation and gas diffusion, *Acta Anaesth. Scand.*, 28, 544, 1984.
80. Isabey, D., Harf, A., and Chang, H. K., Alveolar ventilation during high-frequency oscillation: core dead space concept, *J. Appl. Physiol.*, 56(3), 700, 1984.
81. Scherer, P. W. and Haselton, F. R., Convective exchange in oscillatory flow through bronchial-tree models, *J. Appl. Physiol.*, 53(4), 1023, 1982.
82. Kapitan, S., Hammond, M. D., and West, J. B., Convective interregional mixing during high frequency oscillation (HFO), *Physiologist*, 27 (Abstr.), 244, 1984.
83. Kaiser, K., Davies, N. J. H. Davies, Rodriguez-Roisin, R., and Wagner, P. D., Efficacy of high-frequency ventilation in the presence of extensive $\dot{V}_A/\dot{Q}$ mismatch, *J. Appl. Physiol.*, in press, 1985.
84. Hall, S. M., Strawn, W. B., and Levitzky, M. G., Effect of high-frequency oscillation on blood flow to an atelectatic lung in closed-chest dogs, *Crit. Care Med.*, 12(5), 1984.
85. Kapitan, K., Koga, H., and Wagner, P. D., Effectiveness of high-frequency ventilation (HFV) during unilateral airway obstruction, *Am. Rev. Respir. Dis.*, in press, (Abstr).

Chapter 4

REGULATION OF BREATHING DURING HIGH FREQUENCY VENTILATION

Sandra Jean England

TABLE OF CONTENTS

I. EFFECT OF HFV ON SPONTANEOUS VENTILATION

HFV is used to provide artificial support or supplementation for spontaneous breathing. The effect of the administration of HFV on the timing and depth of spontaneous breaths has, however, received little attention. Several investigators have reported a lengthening of expiratory time, often to the point of apnea, during HFV in animals and humans when complete gas exchange is sustained by the ventilator. Thus it appears that HFV has a profound effect on respiratory control.

Jonzon[1] reported complete inhibition of inspiratory phrenic nerve activity in cats ventilated with HFPPV, but not when either volume triggered or phrenic triggered artificial ventilation was administered. Thompson et al.[2] demonstrated in anesthetized dogs that complete apnea was induced by high frequency oscillation. Similarily England et al.[3] reported apnea with HFOV in anesthetized cats. During short periods of HFOV, Banzett et al.[4] noted that expiratory time was lengthened in anesthetized dogs but complete apnea did not always occur. A CO_2 dependent lengthening of expiratory time has also been reported in anesthetized cats.[5] In the one study[6] of the influence of high frequency oscillation in unanesthetized dogs, apnea or breathing frequencies of less than 3 breathes/min were consistently observed in dogs during quiet wakefulness and quiet sleep.

In infants with RDS, an absence of spontaneous breathing efforts during high frequency oscillation was observed except when they were stimulated by pain or handling.[7] Likewise during high frequency oscillation normal human adult subjects under thiopental anesthesia were also apneic, as were an unanesthetized neonate and an adult with COPD.[8] Carlon et al.[9] using HFJV has reported apnea in patients with respiratory failure when driving pressure was greater than 25 psig. In none of these studies was PCO_2 abnormally low during HFV.

When gas exchange is completely sustained by HFV, no reason for spontaneous ventilatory efforts is apparent. However, it is important to understand the mechanisms by which generation of rhythmic respiratory efforts are inhibited during HFV. In addition to the anecdotal evidence for this inhibition in humans, a series of animal experiments have contributed to an understanding of these mechanisms. These studies have concentrated on afferent pathways known to influence respiratory control.

II. CHEMICAL DRIVE DURING HFV

Kolobow et al.[10] and Phillipson et al.,[11] demonstrated using extra corporeal membrane lungs, that normocarbic apnea was induced in conscious animals when CO_2 was removed by the membrane lung at a rate equal to the animal's rate of CO_2 production. An inhibition of breathing in this situation may occur from removal of breath-by-breath fluctuations in CO_2, which are known to cause variations in carotid chemoreceptor afferent output.[12] An analagous situation may occur with HFV. This reasoning assumes that fluctuating peripheral chemoreceptor output is crucial in sustaining rhythmic respiration, an hypothesis which requires more definite proof. However, for at least two reasons, this cannot be the total explanation for apnea during HFV.

First, during conventional mechanical ventilation gas exchange is adequate and, yet, rhythmic phrenic nerve activity and spontaneous breathing efforts are frequently observed. Second, in anesthetized animals,[2-4] vagotomy dimishes or abolishes the inhibition of inspiration during HFV. This suggests that there is an active inhibition of inspiration during high frequency oscillation. The most likely origin of this inhibition is pulmonary mechanoreceptors.

III. VAGAL AFFERENT ACTIVITIES DURING HFV

Two types of mechanoreceptors with vagal afferents which influence ventilation are found in the trachea and lungs. One type, the pulmonary stretch (slowly adapting) receptors, increase their afferent firing rate in response to increases in lung volume or transpulmonary pressure.[13] The second type, the rapidly adapting or "irritant" receptors, increase their rate of discharge in response to rapid deformations of lung tissue.[13] Both receptor types could be stimulated by the mechanical effects of HFV.

Mean discharge rate of slowly adapting receptors was largely unaffected by HFV in pentobarbital anesthetized cats,[14] although 4 of 9 receptors did fire in relation to the HFV pump stroke. More recent reports,[15,16] however, indicate that during high frequency oscillation the majority of these receptors are entrained to the ventilator. Jonzon[1] has also shown an increase in total vagal afferent activity during HFPPV.

In those studies,[1,16] phrenic nerve activity decreases concomitant with the increase in vagal afferent discharge, presumably due to a reflex inhibition of central inspiratory neuronal discharge. Pack et al.[17] have clearly demonstrated that HFOV during inspiration influences the central timing of this phase of respiration.

However, since lung volume may increase during HFV, caution must be exercised in interpreting these results. Normally, when high frequency oscillation is administered it is accompanied by a constant positive pressure in the circuit. Furthermore, some gas trapping may occur during HFV[18] leading to a further increase in lung volume. The possibility that the increase in pulmonary stretch receptor activity is due solely to a static increase in lung volume is unlikely, since the increase is greater than that observed with increases in lung volume with no superimposed oscillation.[15,16]

Rapidly adapting receptors also increase their firing rate in response to HFOV, although Wozniak et al.[15] found that only half of the studied receptors were entrained to the ventilator and Banzett and Geffroy[14] recorded only 15% entrainment. The latter study has also shown that an increase in activity of rapidly adapting receptors with HFV occurred only at abnormally low lung volumes. As was the case for slowly adapting receptors, HFV induced a greater increase in firing rate of the rapidly adapting receptors than that produced by static shifts in lung volume.[15]

Since HFV decreases central inspiratory activity, and increased afferent discharge of rapidly adapting receptors is believed to be inspiratory promoting, the significance of these changes in rapidly adapting receptor discharge during HFV is unclear. An increase in "irritant" receptor discharge may, however, explain the coughing which has been observed in some conscious dogs with administration of HFV.[24] A decrease in ventilator frequency from 15 Hz to 10 Hz normally alleviates the coughing reaction.

IV. OTHER POSSIBLE SOURCES OF RESPIRATORY INHIBITION DURING HFV

While increased vagal afferent feedback is probably the most potent inhibitory factor to respiration during HFV, activation of other inhibitory pathways may also occur. Thompson et al.[2] noted that 2 of 11 dogs did not re-establish a rhythmic pattern of breathing during HFV following vagotomy. Pursuing the possibility that skeletal muscle spindle afferents, especially those originating in the chest wall, might also have a role, the influence of neuro-muscular blockade on phrenic discharge during HFV was considered.[3] Paralysis with either succinylcholine chloride or pancuronium bromide results in a re-establishment of rhythmic phrenic nerve discharge in apneic dogs during HFV. Furthermore, the combined effect of vagotomy and neuromuscular blockade produced a greater inspiratory output than that resulting from vagotomy alone. It was evident that an increase in vagal activity could re-establish respiratory inhibition since the phrenic activity present following neuromuscular blockade could be abolished by increasing the static lung volume.

However, both this study and that of Banzett et al.[19] investigating the effect of HFV in open chested dogs, do indicate that increased vagal afferent activity can inhibit respiration during HFV when chest wall afferent discharge is greatly diminished or absent.

The inhibitory effect which is eliminated by neuromuscular blockade may result from HFV induced activation of intercostal spindle afferents.[3] Vibration of the chest wall at high frequencies inhibits respiration.[20,21] Neuromuscular blockade is obviously a brute force means of assessing the effects of spindle activation and more detailed studies are required to clarify the effects of HFV on spindle activity.

Only one controlled study involving the effects of HFOV on respiratory inhibition in unanesthetized animals has been reported.[6] In dogs with chronic tracheal stomas, HFOV induced either apnea or near apnea with PCO_2 in the normal range. The most striking aspect of this study was the observation that cessation of spontaneous breathing occurred for prolonged periods (i.e., hours) while the animals were lying quietly awake or were in quiet sleep. However, during phasic rapid eye movement (REM) sleep, spontaneous respiration resumed. This is not surprising since the two postulated inhibitory pathways, vagal[22] and chest wall afferents,[23] are known to be disabled during REM sleep. Spontaneous breathing during bouts of rapid eye movements in infants previously apneic during HFV have been observed,[24] an observation which may well be explained in this manner.

Another interesting, but unexplained, observation is the presence of what appears to be tonic phrenic nerve activity[24] and diaphragmatic[4] activities during the prolonged expiratory phase induced by HFV. It appears that the behavior of the respiratory controller during apnea on HFV may differ from that observed during normal expiration.

V. CONTROVERSIES AND CAVEATS

The effects of HFV on the respiratory control system are not well defined. Even the sparse literature which is available can, and has been, challenged on methological grounds. Thus, there remains a large gap in fundamental understanding, and it can only be eliminated by further experimentation which emphasizes a number of crucial factors. As suggested by Banzett et al.,[4] the effect of HFV per se may well be masked or enhanced by the influences of ventilator settings, changes in lung volume, body temperature, anesthetic agent used coupled with the depth of anesthesia, and blood gases. Each of these variables can alter the output of the respiratory center. In the majority of the experiments cited in this chapter, one or more of these variables has not been controlled.

The term HFV encompasses a diverse collection of ventilator types operated at varying frequencies and delivered volumes. Each ventilator may influence afferent pathways in a different manner. Furthermore, the addition of constant positive pressure which alters lung volume will also effect afferent activity.

It is crucial that blood gases be controlled since the respiratory control system is exquisitely sensitive to changes in chemical homeostasis. Thus, apnea may be induced by HFV more readily if PCO_2 is low and PO_2 is high. Furthermore, anesthetic agents have varying potencies in depressing the respiratory centers and their response to afferent inputs. These effects may enhance or suppress the influence of HFV.

These factors may well account for the discrepancies in published reports on the influence of HFV on the respiratory control system. The difference between the complete apnea observed by some investigators[1-3] and the prolongation of expiratory time observed by others[4,5] may be resolved with a more controlled study of the effects of

HFV per se. Furthermore, the observed activity of vagal afferents is crucially dependent on these factors.

VI. SUMMARY

The use of HFV has profound effects on the respiratory control system. These effects, namely the inhibition of spontaneous, rhythmic inspiratory discharge, are poorly understood. It is obvious, however, that the mechanical effect of HFV leads to an increased afferent discharge of pulmonary mechanoreceptors. Likewise, mechanical influences on the discharge of chest wall mechanoreceptors may also exist. These factors coupled with the artificial support of gas exchange during HFV, appear to provide a potent inhibition of spontaneous inspiration. Evidence also exists that this inhibition is state-dependent, i.e., it is lost during phasic REM sleep.

Inhibition of spontaneous breathing is often desirable during mechanical ventilation. Having a patient "fighting" the ventilator can be deleterious. Conversely, weaning the patient from HFV may be difficult if HFV itself inhibits spontaneous breathing. Therefore, it is important to gain a more thorough understanding of the mechanisms by which the various forms of HFV effect the respiratory control system.

REFERENCES

1. Jonzon, A., Phrenic and vagal nerve activities during spontaneous respiration and positive pressure ventilation, *Acta Anaesth. Scand.*, Suppl. 64, 29, 1977.
2. Thompson, W. K., Marchak, B. E., Bryan, A. C., and Froese, A. B., Vagotomy reverses apnea induced by high frequency oscillatory ventilation, *J. Appl. Physiol.*, 51(6), 1484, 1981.
3. England, S. J., Onayemi, A., and Bryan, A. C., Neuromuscular blockade enhances phrenic nerve activity during high frequency ventilation, *J. Appl. Physiol.*, 56(1), 31, 1984.
4. Banzett, R., Lehr, J., and Geffroy, B., High frequency ventilation lengthens respiration in the anesthetized dog, *J. Appl. Physiol.*, 55(2), 329, 1983.
5. Mautone, A. J., Sica, A. L., and Scarpelli, E. M., Ventilatory control during high frequency oscillation (HFO), *Fed. Proc.*, 41, 1507, 1982.
6. England, S. J., Sullivan, C., Bowes, G., Onayemi, A., and Bryan, A. C., State related alterations of respiration during high frequency ventilation, *Fed. Proc.*, 42(3), 739, 1983.
7. Marchak, B. E., Thompson, W. K., Duffty, P., Miyaki, T., Bryan, M. H., Bryan, A. C., and Froese, A. B., Treatment of RDS by high-frequency oscillatory ventilation: a preliminary report, *J. Pediatr.*, 99, 287, 1981.
8. Butler, W. J., Bohn, D. J., Bryan, A. C., and Froese, A. B., Ventilation by high-frequency oscillation in humans, *Anesth. Analg.*, 59(8), 577, 1980.
9. Carlon, G. C., Kahn, R. C., Howland, W. S., Ray, C., Jr., and Turnbull, A. D., Clinical experience with high frequency jet ventilation, *Crit. Care Med.*, 9(1), 1, 1981.
10. Kolobow, T., Gattinoni, L., Tomlinson, T. A., and Pierce, J. E., Control of breathing using an extracorporeal membrane lung, *Anesthesiology*, 46, 138, 1977.
11. Phillipson, E. A., Duffin, J., and Cooper, J. D., Critical dependence of respiratory rhythmicity on metabolic CO_2 load, *J. Appl. Physiol.*, 50, 45, 1981.
12. Briscoe, T. J. and Willshaw, P., Stimulus-response relationships of the peripheral arterial chemoreceptors, in *Regulation of Breathing*, Part 1, Hornbein, T. F., Ed., Marcel Dekker, New York, 1981, 321.
13. Widdicombe, J. G., Nervous receptors in the respiratory tract and lungs, in *Regulation of Breathing*, Part 1, Hornbein, T. F., Ed., Marcel Dekker, New York, 1981, 429.
14. Banzett, R. B. and Geffroy, B., Response of cat pulmonary receptors to high frequency oscillation, *Fed. Proc.*, 41, 988, 1982.
15. Wozniak, J. A., Davenport, P. W., and Kosch, P. C., The response of pulmonary afferents to high frequency oscillatory ventilation, *Fed. Proc.*, 43, 1016, 1983.

16. Man, G. C. W., Man, S. F. P., and Kappagoda, C. T., Effects of high frequency oscillatory ventilation on vagal and phrenic nerve activities, *J. Appl. Physiol.*, 54(2), 502, 1983.
17. Pack, A. I., Davies, R. O., Marino, P. L., and Fishman, A. P., Effects of high frequency oscillatory air flow on control of inspiratory duration, *Fed. Proc.*, 39, 1075, 1980.
18. Saari, A. F., Rossing, T. H., Solway, J., and Drazen, J. M., Lung inflation during high frequency ventilation, *Am. Rev. Respir. Dis.*, 129, 333, 1984.
19. Banzett, R., Reid, M., and Lehr, J., High frequency oscillation of the lung alone lengthens expiration in anesthetized dogs, *Fed. Proc.*, 43, 814, 1984.
20. Homma, I., Inspiratory inhibitory reflex caused by the chest wall vibration in man, *Respir. Physiol.*, 39, 345, 1980.
21. Remmers, J. E., Inhibition of inspiratory activity by intercostal muscle afferents, *Respir. Physiol.*, 10, 358, 1970.
22. Sullivan, C. E., Murphy, E., Kozar, L. F., and Phillipson, E. A., Ventilatory responses to CO_2 and lung inflation in tonic versus phasic REM sleep, *J. Appl. Physiol.*, 47, 1304, 1979.
23. Gassel, M. M. and Pompeiano, O., An analysis of the supraspinal influences acting on motoneurones during sleep in the unrestrained cat. Modification of the recurrent discharge of the alpha motoneurones during sleep, *Arch. Ital. Biol.*, 103, 347, 1965.
24. England, S. J., Unpublished observation.

Chapter 5

HIGH FREQUENCY VENTILATION BY TRANSTHORACIC OSCILLATION

H. K. Chang

TABLE OF CONTENTS

I. INTRODUCTION

While the majority of studies on HFV are devoted to HFJV or HFOV,[1-3] a different method involving transthoracic oscillation has demonstrated distinct advantages. Even before the development of HFV in the late 1960s, ventilation by transthoracic oscillation had been used widely for several decades.[4] The most notable devices of this type of mechanical ventilation were the Drinker Respirator or "Iron Lung"[5] and Cuirass Respirators.[6] These devices applied alternating negative and positive pressure either to the whole body surface excluding the head or to the thoracoabdominal surface, generating breaths of comparable frequency and tidal volume to those found in spontaneous breathing. These respirators were used mainly in chronic care for patients suffering from muscle paralysis, and were gradually replaced by the intermittent positive pressure ventilators of the 1950s.

As the concept of low-volume HFV began to attract the interest of investigators in the early 1980s, it seemed logical to combine the older concept of transthoracic ventilation with the newer concept of HFV.

The first application of transthoracic HFV was performed in Montreal in 1981. Zidulka et al.[7] compressed the dog's thorax at frequencies from 3 to 11 Hz (180 to 660 c/min) by means of an air-filled cuff attached around the animal and a reciprocating air pump. Except that the pressure in the cuff remained above atmospheric at all times, this method of HFV resembled the Cuirass respirator in its basic configuration.

Extending this application, Harf et al.[8] ventilated apneic rats in a body-chamber by oscillating the air pressure in the chamber at 20 Hz (1200 c/min). Ward et al.[9] used the same principle to ventilate spontaneously breathing cats at frequencies between 0.5 and 30 Hz. Piquet et al.[10] applied this method in apneic rabbits and obtained good oxygenation and normocapnia at 1 to 16 Hz. In these three applications the experimental animals (rats, cats, rabbits) had tracheostomies, with their entire bodies placed inside the chamber. Envisaging eventual use of this method in infants, Chartrand et al.[11] adopted a configuration similar to the Drinker respirator and to a later version for infants known as Isolette Respirator (Airshields Inc., Hatboro, Pa.).[12] These workers successfully ventilated, at 3 to 15 Hz, apneic as well as spontaneously breathing rabbits whose heads remained outside the body chamber.

The method of transthoracic HFV has also been applied to spontaneously breathing, awake man, both in the sitting[13] and supine[14] position. The results indicated that this technique reduced spontaneous minute ventilation and/or increased alveolar ventilation.

Unforseen by the early researchers in HFV, transthoracic HFV above a certain minimum frequency has been shown[15-17] also to enhance mucus clearance from the lung. Thus, the advent of HFV has given the Iron Lung and the Cuirass respirators not only a new dimension in terms of higher frequency but also a new purpose as a form of chest physiotherapy.

II. TYPES OF APPARATUS AND APPLICATIONS

There are basically two types of transthoracic HFV. One involves only the thoracic surface. The other utilizes the entire body surface (sometimes excepting the head).

The first type is known as HFCWO and employs a cuff or a vest around the thorax of the subject (Figure 1). Air is delivered into and withdrawn from this device by a reciprocating pump at a preset amplitude and frequency. The efficiency of this apparatus depends on the area of apposition between the cuff and the chest wall, as well as on the mean pressure in the cuff. This basic construct has been employed by Zidulka et al.,[7] Gross et al.,[17,18] and King et al.[15,16] with dogs and Calverley et al.[14] and Harf et al.[13] with man.

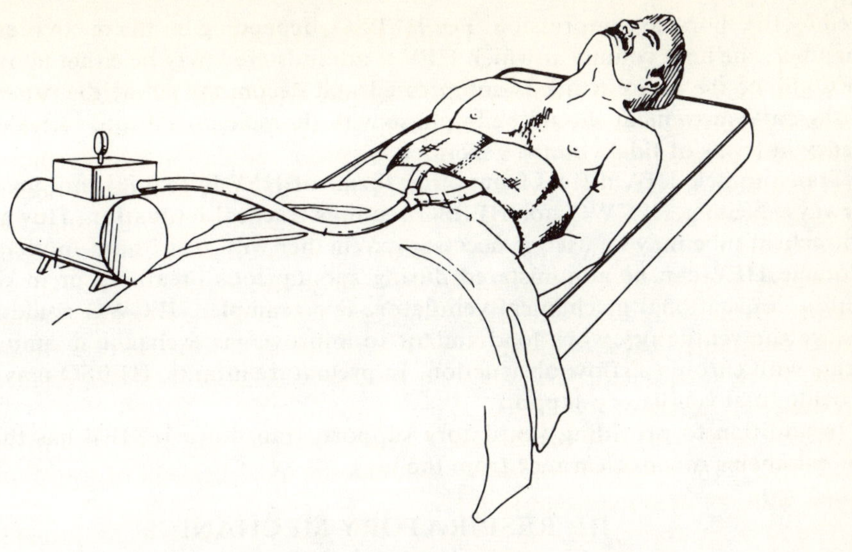

FIGURE 1. A sketch of the apparatus used in HFCWO.

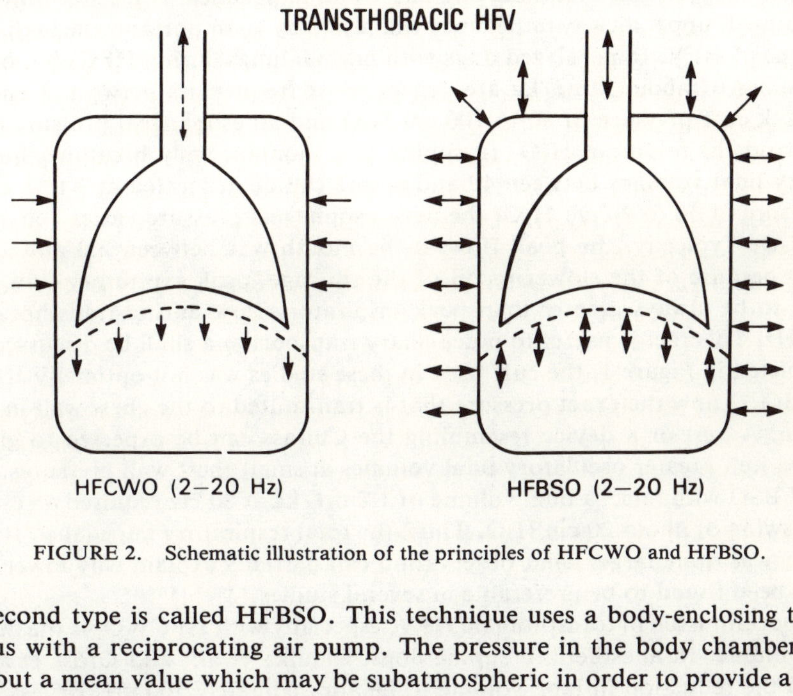

FIGURE 2. Schematic illustration of the principles of HFCWO and HFBSO.

The second type is called HFBSO. This technique uses a body-enclosing tank-type apparatus with a reciprocating air pump. The pressure in the body chamber is oscillated about a mean value which may be subatmospheric in order to provide a constant airway distending pressure. For reasons of energy requirement, this apparatus is best suited for small infants. At the present time, no human subjects have been ventilated by HFBSO. However, it has been used by Harf et al.[8] with rats, Ward et al.[9] with cats, and by Piquet et al.[10] and Chartrand et al.[11] with rabbits.

The basic concepts and the mechanical actions of transthoracic HFV are shown schematically in Figure 2. For HFCWO, expiration is caused by chest wall compression and inspiration results from passive recoil of the chest wall. The tidal breaths are inspired at a lung volume just below functional residual capacity (FRC). If nothing is used to prevent the movement of the abdominal content, the diaphragm tends to descend as the thoracic cage is compressed, thus dissipating the alveolar pressure generated by the thoracic compression. For HFBSO, depending on the mean pressure in the chamber, the lung volume at which HFV is administered may be either above or below FRC. Since the entire trunk is compressed and decompressed at the same time, diaphragmatic movement should be in phase with thoracic oscillation, increasing its efficiency in terms of tidal volume generated.

Transthoracic HFV differs from other forms of HFV in that it is not invasive to the airways. Neither HFCWO nor HFBSO requires tracheal intubation. However, an endotracheal tube may be used if necessary. Whether with or without intubation, transthoracic HFV can be administered during spontaneous breathing or in conjunction with a conventional mechanical ventilator. For example, HFCWO could be used to reduce the ventilatory work load and/or to improve gas exchange in ambulatory patients with chronic airflow obstruction. In premature infants, HFBSO may be used to provide total ventilatory support.

In addition to providing ventilatory support, transthoracic HFV has the potential for enhancing mucus clearance from the lung.

III. RESPIRATORY MECHANICS

Since transthoracic HFV produces tidal breaths by compressing the thoracic cage, its efficiency depends on both lung and chest wall impedance. If tracheal intubation is not performed, upper airway impedance will also play an important role in the efficacy of this type of HFV. In paralyzed dogs with normal lungs during HFCWO, oscillatory tidal volumes of about 2 mℓ/kg are generated at frequencies between 3 and 11 Hz, with a peak cuff pressure of 80 to 100 cm H_2O and an esophageal pressure excursion ranging from 10 to 20 cm H_2O. In supine and spontaneously breathing humans[13,14] oscillatory tidal volumes between 40 and 60 mℓ can be generated at 3 to 8 Hz with a cuff pressure of 50 to 90 cm H_2O; the peak esophageal pressure varies between 8 and 13 cm H_2O. Typically, the peak flow at the mouth was between 2.0 and 2.5 ℓ/sec. Probably because of the slower recoil of the rib cage, peak expiratory flow has been observed to be always greater than peak inspiratory flow during transthoracic HFV above 3 Hz. This fact is useful to mucociliary transport and shall be discussed later.

As depicted in Figure 1, the cuff used in these studies was not optimally efficient. It is difficult to know the exact pressure that is transmitted to the chest wall in this configuration. A vest or a device resembling the Cuirass can be expected to give better efficiency, i.e., greater oscillatory tidal volumes at small chest wall pressures.

For HFBSO with rats,[8] a tidal volume of 1.9 mℓ/kg at 20 Hz required an esophageal pressure swing of about 20 cm H_2O. Thus, the total respiratory impedance at this high frequency was quite large. That observation can partially explain why lower frequencies have been found to be preferable in several studies.[7,10,11,14,18,19]

An important issue in transthoracic HFV, especially with HFCWO, is the depression of lung volume. In anesthetized supine dogs, Zidulka et al.[7] and Gross et al.[18] both estimated the reduction in lung volume to be approximately 100 mℓ, or less than 5% of FRC. In awake supine humans, the reduction in FRC was found by Calverley et al.[14] to vary between 200 and 300 mℓ. In sitting man, Harf et al.[8] estimated the change in FRC to be near 125 and 200 mℓ at an oscillatory tidal volume of 20 and 40 mℓ, respectively. Again, these changes were less than 5% of the average FRC of the subjects studied.

Similar estimates have not been made during HFBSO, but they can be expected to not exceed 5% of FRC when the mean chamber pressure is atmospheric. In the case of a negative mean pressure in the chamber, the operating range of HFBSO should be equal to or greater than FRC.

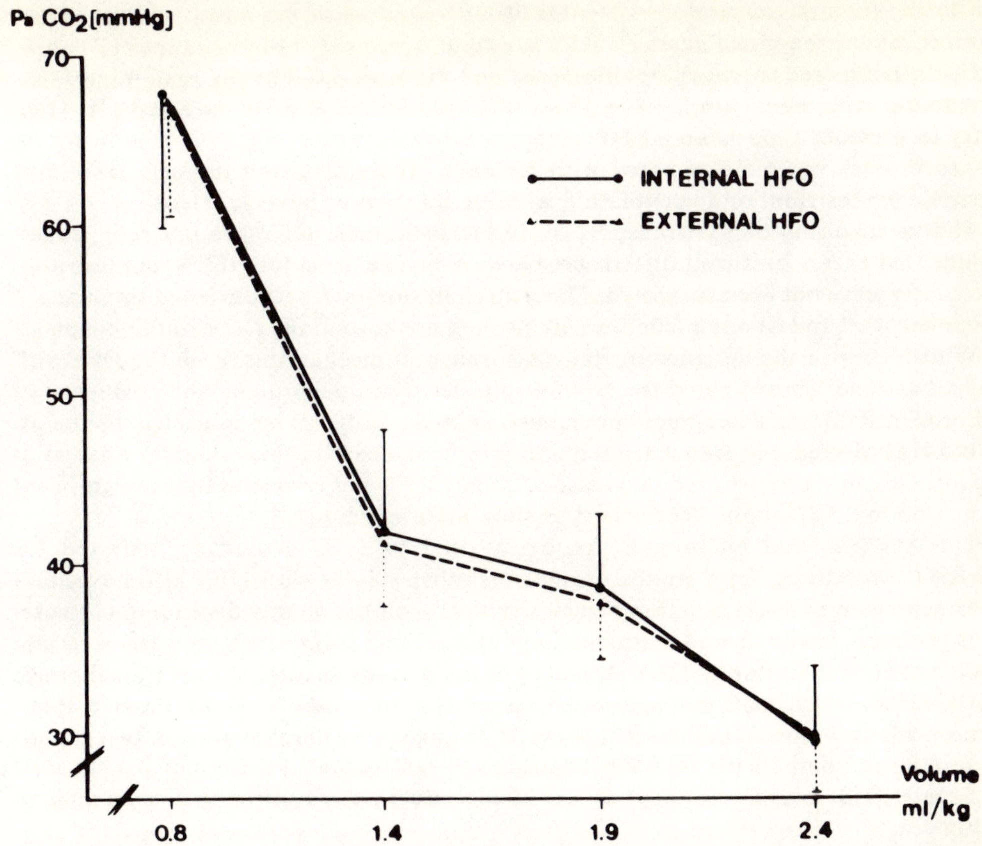

FIGURE 3. Comparison of arterial CO_2 pressure during HFBSO (external HFOV) and HFOV (internal HFOV) in relation to magnitude of the oscillation.

IV. GAS EXCHANGE

Despite a possible slight depression of resting lung volume, transthoracic HFV has been shown to allow adequate gas exchange in paralyzed normal rats, rabbits, and dogs and to enhance alveolar ventilation in spontaneously breathing cats, rabbits, dogs, and humans. Unlike HFJV and HFOV, which have been found to be rather ineffective in obstructive lung disease,[3] transthoracic HFV appears to improve gas exchange in the presence of airway obstruction.[18,19]

In paralyzed dogs, Zidulka et al.[7] found that HFCWO at 5 Hz with a total volume of 2.5 mℓ/kg yielded stable arterial oxygen pressure (Pa_{O_2}) greater than 80 mm Hg and arterial carbon dioxide pressure (Pa_{CO_2}) less than 30 mm Hg. At 11 Hz and with a tidal volume of less than 2 mℓ/kg, adequate gas exchange could not be maintained in the same dogs, apparently because of the decrease in tidal volume.

To compare the gas exchange efficacy of HFBSO and HFOV, Harf et al.[8] applied the same tidal volumes and frequencies to the same group of rats and measured similar blood gases. Figure 3 shows the Pa_{CO_2} as a function of tidal volume when the frequency was fixed at 20 Hz for both HFOV (internal HFO) and HFBSO (external HFO). It is thus evident that the two types of transthoracic HFV, i.e., HFCWO and HFBSO, are not only adequate but also as effective as HFOV in promoting pulmonary gas exchange, at least in the normal lung.

Picquet et al.[19] induced bronchoconstriction on apneic rabbits ventilated with

HFBSO. When the respiratory system resistances increased three- to fivefold over the control values, the blood gases were improved at 5 Hz with a tidal volume of 1.5 mℓ/kg when compared to the values measured at 1 Hz with a tidal volume of 4.0 mℓ/kg. The rate of CO_2 elimination was also significantly higher at 5 Hz than at 1 Hz. Contrary to previous reports about HFOV applied to obstructed lungs, no significant increase in lung volume was noted with HFBSO. Therefore, transthoracic HFV may decrease maldistribution in ventilation without appreciable adverse effects.

The mechanisms of gas transport during transthoracic HFV are not fully understood. However, significant differences between mechanisms for HFOV and transthoracic HFV have not been suspected. These mechanisms have been reviewed by Chang,[20] Kamm et al.,[21] and Chapter 2 in this volume, and are beyond the scope of this chapter.

While not specially designed to study gas transport mechanisms, both Piquet et al.[10] and Chartrand[11] investigated the relationship between tidal volume and frequency of HFBSO in stable normocapnic experimental animals. Both studies indicated that below 5 to 6 Hz a decrease in frequency requires a large increase in tidal volume, whereas at frequencies above 6 to 8 Hz an increase of frequency is not rewarded by any significant reduction in tidal volume necessary to maintain normocapnia.

This suggests that an optimal frequency of 5 to 6 Hz should be preferred for HFBSO. Moreover, these studies suggest, as other studies with HFV also have, that satisfactory arterial oxygenation depends critically on the airway distending pressure. This probably results from the smaller lung volume excursion which produces a certain degree of atelectasis during HFV. Whether or not atelectasis exists during transthoracic HFV, arterial oxygenation is generally less satisfactory than is carbon dioxide elimination. Figure 4 shows the plots of V_T vs. f during stable normocapnia in two groups of rabbits ventilated with HFBSO, at either a mean tracheal pressure of 0.5 cm H_2O or 5 cm H_2O. It is apparent that CO_2 elimination does not significantly depend on lung volume.

Transthoracic HFV has the advantage that it can be combined with spontaneous breathing. In normal supine man, HFCWO at 3 and 5 Hz resulted in decreases in spontaneous minute ventilation averaging 25 and 35%, respectively.[14] By contrast, the blood gas tensions in these subjects remained essentially unchanged with or without the superimposed HFCWO. When the spontaneous breathing frequency and tidal volume were regulated,[13] superimposed HFCWO at 5 Hz and a moderate tidal volume resulted in much faster (by 25%) nitrogen washouts than spontaneous breathing alone. This occurred despite a decrease of lung volume by 5% during HFCWO. Harf et al.[13] postulated that this was due to enhanced gas mixing in the lung periphery during the inspiratory phase of spontaneous breathing and improved gas mixing in the airways during spontaneous expiration. Whatever the precise reasons for the faster washouts, this study was complimentary to that of Calverley et al.[14] cited above, and demonstrated improved alveolar ventilation by the superimposed HFCWO.

V. MUCOCILIARY TRANSPORT

Since percussion is a standard form of chest physiotherapy and commercial vibrators promoting mucus clearance in patients suffering from obstructive and fibrotic lung diseases already exist, it is logical that transthoracic HFV, at least HFCWO at certain frequencies, could also enhance mucus clearance from the lung. In fact, Beck[22] in 1966 reported the use of a device similar to the apparatus depicted in Figure 1 to help patients with obstructive lung disease to expectorate. However, these results were unknown to Zidulka et al.[7] during their initial experiments with HFCWO. The possibility of HFCWO enhancing mucociliary transport was not apparent until they observed that peak expiratory flowrate was systematically greater than the peak inspiratory flowrate.

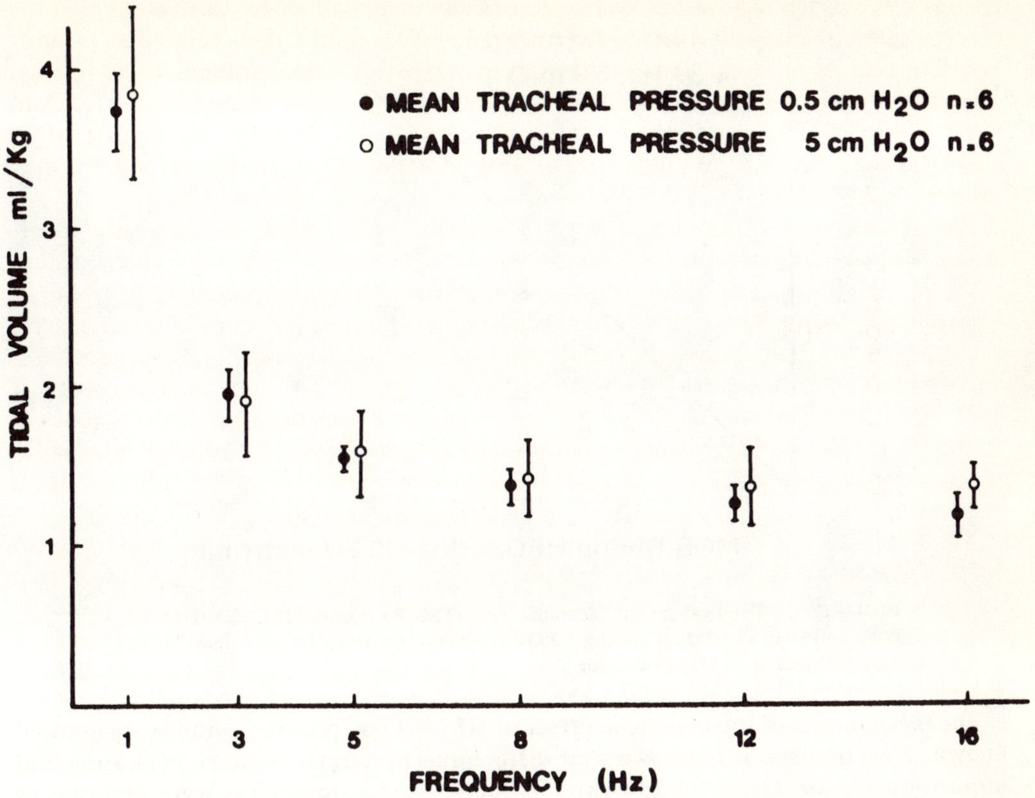

FIGURE 4. Comparison of tidal volumes necessary to maintain stable normocapnia in rabbits ventilated with HFBSO; the mean tracheal pressure for one group (n = 6) was 0.5 cm H_2O, for the other group (n = 6) it was 5.0 cm H_2O.

They reasoned that if directional air-mucus shearing is a valid mechanism of mucus or sputum clearance, as it is in coughing, then HFCWO should result in an enhanced mouthward movement of mucus because of the cumulative effect of a greater expiratory flow rate in each oscillatory cycle.

King et al.[15,16] confirmed this reasoning in a convincing manner. Applying HFCWO at 3 to 17 Hz to anesthetized dogs and producing oscillatory tidal volumes of 25 to 100 mℓ, at all frequencies above 3 Hz the tracheal mucus clearance rate (TMCR) was increased over baseline TMCR determined during spontaneous breathing. The enhancement was most pronounced in the range of 11 to 15 Hz, reaching a peak value of 340% of control at 13 Hz. In a follow-up study, the TMCR in anesthetized dogs during spontaneous breathing (SB) was compared during HFCWO and HFOV. At 13 Hz with an oscillatory tidal volume of 1.5 mℓ/kg, mean TMCR was 240% of control with HFCWO and 76% of control with HFOV. McEvoy et al.[23] had earlier reported that HFOV might adversely affect mucociliary transport. To repeat the conditions studied by the latter authors, King et al. also applied HFOV at 20 Hz. Figure 5 shows an identity plot of TMCR during HFCWO at 13 Hz against HFOV at 13 and 20 Hz. It is clear that HFCWO at 13 Hz produced significantly greater mucus clearance than HFOV. Using a radioisotope and a gamma camera to determine regional lung clearance and determining the transport rate of a tracheal marker by bronchoscopic visualization, as did King et al.,[15,16] Gross et al.[17] reported that HFCWO is effective in enhancing both peripheral and central mucus clearance in dogs. Furthermore, the method was determined to be safe when moderate pressures were applied.

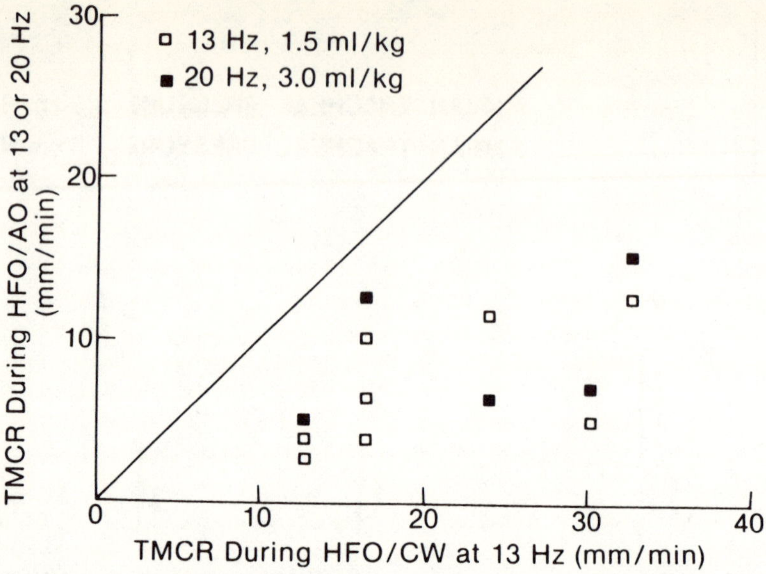

FIGURE 5. Tracheal mucus clearance rate (TMCR) during HFCWO (HFOV/CW) at 13 Hz vs. TMCR during HFOV (HFOV/AO) at 13 Hz with same V_T as HFCWO and at 20 Hz at twice the V_T.

The mechanisms of the beneficial effect of HFCWO on mucus clearance are not well known. Nevertheless, it is known that differential flow rates between expiration and inspiration during HFCWO can produce biased shear forces favoring mouthward movement of mucus. In an in vitro experiment and a theoretical model, Chang et al.[24] demonstrated that the velocity of mucus movement is proportional to $\delta V_T f^{1.5}$ (R-1), where δ is thickness of the mucus layer; V_T is tidal volume; f is frequency; and R is the ratio of peak expiratory flow rate to peak inspiratory flow rate. Since R has been found to be greater than unity in animal experiments with all HFCWO studies to date and with an HFBSO study in rabbits, it is likely that both forms of transthoracic HFV will always have a positive effect on mucus clearance.

Whether differential shearing at the air-mucus interface is the only, or the dominant, mechanism is uncertain. King et al.[25] examined this by comparing TMCR during HFCWO with its intrinsic expiratory flow rate bias and during HFOV maneuvers were not as effective as the HFCWO maneuvers, indicating that a flow rate bias is not the only, or even the dominant, mechanism for the observed enhancement of TMCR. Vagal stimulation of ciliary beating via afferent receptors may also play a role.

Regardless the physiological mechanisms involved, the use of transthoracic HFV in human patients is worth considering. Since the best frequency for gas exchange appears to be about 6 Hz, and for mucociliary transport about 13 Hz, it is doubtful whether the same device can be used advantageously for both purposes simultaneously.

VI. CARDIOVASCULAR FUNCTION

Two questions may be asked concerning the effect of transthoracic HFV on cardiovascular function. First, does the use of transthoracic HFV cause serious derangements in the cardiovascular performance? Second, can transthoracic HFV be used as a form of cardiac resuscitation? Currently, no firm and complete answer can be given to either question, but the existing evidence suggests a negative answer to the first question and possibly an affirmative answer to the sescond question.

In spontaneously breathing dogs with and without superimposed HFCWO at 3, 5, and 8 Hz, Gross et al.[18] measured cardiac output, systemic blood pressure, central venous pressure, pulmonary artery, and wedge pressures; they found no significant difference in any of these variables. Similar studies have not been made to date when HFCWO alone was used to maintain gas exchange.

With HFBSO, several investigations[9,11,19] have reported stable heart rate, mean arterial pressure, and central venous pressure except in the presence of hypercapnia or severe respiratory acidosis. The frequencies used in these studies range from 1 to 30 Hz and the tidal volumes from 1.5 to 4.0 mℓ/kg. Though additional work, especially direct measurement of cardiac output, is needed, it appears that transthoracic HFV does not impede venous return or cardiac output. Moreover, despite its compression on the thoraco-abdominal surface, HFBSO has little or no effect on other hemodynamic parameters.[11]

When the head is outside the body chamber and a neck seal is used in HFBSO, there is a possibility that cerebral blood flow may be influenced; this is an area for further investigations.

Chartrand et al.[11] made simultaneous recordings of arterial pressure, central venous pressure, and esophageal pressure in rabbits before, during, and after ventilation with HFBSO. The shape of the esophageal pressure tracing was considered to be an accurate reflection of the body chamber pressure variation. With HFBSO, the arterial pressure profile became highly irregular so that systolic and diastolic phases could not be distinguished. However, by subtracting the esophageal pressure signal from the deranged arterial pressure signal, one could recover an arterial pressure tracing almost identical to that recorded during SB alone. This suggests that the pressure variations at the body surface are accurately transmitted through the chest wall, and the intrapleural pressure changes are easily and accurately transmitted through the vascular wall. This observation leaves open the possibility of using HFBSO as a means of cardiac assist by counter pulsation.

Indeed, in the earlier application of the Cuirass respirator, Eisenmenger[6] demonstrated the possibility of cardiac resuscitation with this device. Working with HFJV, Carlon et al.[26] suggested that increasing transmural aortic pressure by increasing airway pressure during systolic ejection aids left ventricular emptying. Based on the evidence presented above, it seems that timing peak compressing pressure during HFBSO or HFCWO with a certain event in the cardiac cycle could also enhance cardiac performance. This aspect of transthoracic HFV has not been investigated, but appears to be very attractive.

VII. CONTROL OF BREATHING

Though many researchers have reported episodes of apnea when HFV of any form is applied only very scanty critical data have been presented in terms of ventilatory control. With transthoracic HFV superimposed on SB, two occurrences have been cited.

Gross et al.[18] observed a significant reduction in spontaneous minute ventilation in dogs during HFCWC, with the reduction mainly a result of a decrease in tidal volume. The reasons for this particular pattern of breathing are not clear. Calverley et al.[14] found a reduction in minute ventilation of up to 40% in awake normal humans during HFCWC. The arterial P_{CO_2} of these subjects remained constant despite large decreases in minute ventilation. A likely explanation for this phenomenon is that the amount of spontaneous minute ventilation is regulated centrally to sufficiently maintain a constant arterial P_{CO_2}. When an efficient gas transport process is introduced by HFCWO, more CO_2 must be eliminated per breath, hence the decrease in minute ventilation.

The seond type of data concerns apnea, which occurred in some dogs studied by Gross et al.[18] with HFCWO and in cats studied by Ward et al.[9] with HFBSO. Even though central regulation of P_{CO_2} may be a reason for this occurrence, a reflex mechanism mediated by receptors in the chest wall is also a likely possibility. England et al.[28] reported that rhythmic phrenic discharge disappeared during HFOV in cats at normal levels of Pa_{CO_2}, but the phrenic activity returned after neuromuscular blockade in the vagally intact animal. Although vagotomy alone also restored phrenic discharge, this activity was further enhanced by neuromuscular blockade. Thus, it appears that apnea during HFV results from inspiratory inhibition mediated by both chest wall and vagal afferent mechanisms. Clearly, a greater understanding of the mechanisms of control of breathing during transthoracic HFV will have important ramifications in its eventual adoption as a form of ventilatory assist.

VIII. SAFETY CONSIDERATIONS

Since transthoracic HFV is intended for eventual clinical use, the safety must first be established. The existing data appear to be encouraging in this regard.

No adverse disturbances in the cardiovascular function have been observed.[11,14,18] Upon autopsy of dogs ventilated with HFCWO, no pneuncothorax and only minimal local atelactasis has been found.[7,18] Serum hemoglobin and creatine phosphokinase (CPK) values did not change after prolonged HFCWO in both dogs[18] and man.[14]

The safety features of HFBSO have been less well documented. At least two relevant points need to be considered in detail: (1) the influence of the neck seal on cerebral blood flow; and (2) possible aeration of the gastrointestinal tract due to the negative chamber pressure.

Since transthoracic HFV is still at the experimental stage, its neurological effects have not been but should definitely be investigated.

IX. CONCLUSION

There now exists two forms of transthoracic HFV, neither requires invasion of the airways. Operated below 10 Hz, HFCWO allows adequate gas exchange in apneic subjects and reduces minute ventilation in spontaneously breathing subjects. At 10 Hz or above, it appears to enhance mucus clearance from the lung. The body-enclosing type HFBSO is better suited for smaller subjects, both to provide ventilatory support and possibly as a form of cardiac assist.

Although additional research is required, transthoracic HFV may be potentially useful in at least three clinical applications:

1. HFCWO as partial ventilatory support in ambulatory patients
2. HFBSO in neonatal critical care
3. Both HFCWO and HFBSO as a form of chest physiotherapy

REFERENCES

1. Smith, R. B., Ventilation at high respiratory frequencies, *Anaesthesia*, 37, 1011, 1982.
2. Drazen, J. M., Kamm, R. D., and Slutsky, A. S., High-frequency ventilation, *Physiol. Rev.*, 64, 505, 1984.
3. Chang, H. K. and Harf, A., High-frequency ventilation: a review, *Respir. Physiol.*, 57, 135, 1984.

4. Woollam, C. H. M., The development of apparatus for intermittent negative pressure respiration, *Anaesthesia,* 31, 666, 1976.
5. Drinker, P. and McKhann, C. F., The use of a new apparatus for the prolonged administration of artificial respiration, *J. Am. Med. Assoc.,* 92, 1658, 1929.
6. Eisenmenger, R., Therapeutic application of supra-abdominal suction and compressed air in relation to respiration and circulation, *Wien. Med. Wochenschr.,* 89, 1032, 1939.
7. Zidulka, A., Gross, D., Minami, H., Vartian, V., and Chang, H. K., Ventilation by high-frequency chest wall compression in dogs with normal lungs, *Am. Rev. Respir. Dis.,* 127, 709, 1983.
8. Harf, A., Bertrand, C., and Chang, H. K., Ventilation by high-frequency oscillation of thorax or at trachea in rats, *J. Appl. Physiol.,* 56, 155, 1984.
9. Ward, H. E., Armengal, J., and Jones, R. L., Ventilation by external high-frequency oscillation in cats, *Chest,* 82 (Abstr), 211, 1982.
10. Piquet, J., Isabey, D., Chang, H. K., and Harf, A., Stable normocapnia during high-frequency body-surface oscillation in rabbits, *Am. Rev. Respir. Dis.,* 132, 104, 1985.
11. Chartrand, D., Phillips, D. M., Sun, R., Harf, A., and Chang, H. K., Ventilation by high-frequency body-surface oscillation in normal rabbits, *Clin. Resp. Physiol.,* submitted for publication.
12. Outerbridge, E. W. and Stern, L., Negative pressure ventilators, in *Assisted Ventilation of the Neonate,* Goldsmith, J. P. and Karotkin, E. K., Eds., W. B. Saunders, Philadelphia, 1981, chap. 8.
13. Harf, A., Zidulka, A., and Chang, H. K., Nitrogen washout during tidal breathing with superimposed high frequency chest wall oscillation, *Am. Rev. Respir. Dis.,* 132, 350, 1985.
14. Calverley, P. M. A., Chang, H. K., Vartian, V., and Ziculka, A., High frequency chest wall oscillation: assistance to ventilation in spontaneously breathing subjects, *Chest,* 89, 218, 1986.
15. King, M., Phillips, D. M., Gross, D., Vartian, V., Chang, H. K., and Zidulka, A., Enhanced tracheal mucus clearance with high frequency chest wall compression, *Am. Rev. Respir. Dis.,* 128, 511, 1983.
16. King, M., Phillips, D. M., Zidulka, A., and Chang, H. K., Tracheal mucus clearance in high-frequency oscillation. II. Chest wall versus mouth oscillation, *Am. Rev. Respir. Dis.,* 130, 703, 1984.
17. Gross, D., O'Brien, C., Wight, D., Rosenthall, L., Zidulka, A., and King, M., Enhanced peripheral mucus clearance with high frequency chest wall compression, *Physiologist,* 26, A35, 1983.
18. Gross, D., Vartian, V., Minami, H., Chang, H. K., and Zidulka, A., High-frequency chest wall compression aids CO_2 elimination in obstructed dogs, *Clin. Resp. Physiol.,* 20, 507, 1984.
19. Piquet, J., Isabey, D., Chang, H. K., and Harf, A., High frequency transthoracic ventilation improves gas exchange during experimental bronchoconstriction, *Am. Rev. Respir. Dis.,* in press.
20. Chang, H. K., Mechanisms of gas transport during ventilation by high frequency oscillation, *J. Appl. Physiol.,* 56, 553, 1984.
21. Kamm, R. D., Slutsky, A. S., and Drazen, J. M., High-frequency ventilation, *CRC Crit. Rev. Biomed. Eng.,* 9, 347, 1984.
22. Beck, G. J., Chronic bronchial asthma and emphysema rehabilitation and use of thoracic vibrocompression, *Geriatrics,* 21, 139, 1966.
23. McEvoy, R. D., Davies, N. J. H., Hedenstierna, G., Hartman, M. T., Spragg, R. G., and Wagner, P. D., Lung mucociliary transport during high-frequency ventilation, *Am. Rev. Respir. Dis.,* 126, 452, 1982a.
24. Chang, H. K., Weber, M. E., and King, M., Mucus transport by high frequency non-symmetrical oscillatory air flow, *J. Appl. Physiol.,* submitted.
25. King, M., Zidulka, A., Phillips, D. M., Wight, D., Gross, D., and Chang, H. K., Tracheal mucus clearance in high frequency oscillation: effect of peak flow rate bias, *J. Appl. Physiol.,* submitted.
26. Carlon, G. C., Pierri, M. K., Ray, C., Jr., and Kvetan, V., Hemodynamic and respiratory variables with high frequency jet ventilation (HFJV) synchronized with heart rate, *Crit. Care Med.,* 9, 163, 1981.
27. Phillipson, E. A., Duffin, J., and Cooper, J. D., Critical dependence of respiratory rhythmicity on metabolic CO_2 load, *J. Appl. Physiol.,* 50, 45, 1981.
28. England, S. J., Onayemi, A., and Bryan, A. C., Neuromuscular blockade enhances phrenic nerve activity during high-frequency ventilation, *J. Appl. Physiol.,* 56, 31, 1984.

Chapter 6

HEMODYNAMIC EFFECTS OF HIGH FREQUENCY VENTILATION

Erik A. Hagen, Richard L. Bucciarelli, and Josef Neu

TABLE OF CONTENTS

I. INTRODUCTION

Mechanical ventilation, whether at high frequencies or conventional rates, relies on the creation of a positive pressure wave (i.e., tidal volume) that is introduced into the patient's airway via an endotracheal tube. This pressure wave has the potential to directly affect intrathoracic structures that are sensitive to pressure changes. With mechanical ventilation, the alveolus is the structure one aims to reach, but the nature of thoracic anatomy unavoidably exposes pulmonary vasculature and all intrathoracic structures that are pressure-sensitive.

II. BACKGROUND

As with many other advances in the medical sciences, the earliest studies of HFV did not focus on direct medical applications. Henderson's et al.[1] studies in the early 1900s, were intended to investigate a basic physiological phenomenon, i.e., the dead space of the lung. Some of the other early studies investigated interactions between the cardiovascular system and the lung. Using a piston pump, Lunkenheimer et al.[2-4] applied oscillations to the airways of paralyzed dogs so they could study various cardiac phenomena without interference by lungs moving over their field of observation during mechanical inflations and deflations. These investigators observed that at frequencies between 23 and 40 Hz, PaO_2 and $PaCO_2$ remained at normal levels. Contrary to the positive pulmonary effects, the animals showed cardiovascular compromise by developing metabolic acidosis, declining blood pressure, and oliguria. These deleterious cardiovascular changes may have discouraged the investigators from pursuing high frequency oscillation further as a treatment modality for patients with respiratory compromise.

Other investigators, not directly involved in studies of HFV, but with an interest in cardiac-pulmonary interactions, laid some of the important groundwork that stimulated its later clinical application. Fukuchi et al.[5] established that when motion of the beating heart is transmitted to the surrounding lung, gas diffusion is enhanced — a phenomenon known as cardiogenic mixing. Using eight dogs, these investigators measured a 5.59-fold increase in the effective diffusivity of gas in bronchioles which were 2.5 to 8.6 mm in diameter. They attributed this to the transmitted impetus of cardiac contraction. Butler et al.[6] postulated that this phenomenon could be exploited in humans by providing a more energetic "mixer". Using a loudspeaker as their mixer, they directed its output into large bore tubing attached to the human subjects and a capnograph and found that CO_2 "poured out" when the loudspeaker cycled a displacement of 60 mℓ (less than the volume of physiological dead space) at 5 Hz. Bohn et al.[7] subsequently studied the technique in an animal model using a piston-pump device. They found that the optimal frequency for CO_2 elimination in their dogs was 15 Hz at a tidal volume of 1.9 mℓ/kg. In these experiments, cardiac output of the animals did not fall and metabolic acidosis did not develop. The investigators then studied the technique further in patients with respiratory failure.

About a decade before the reports of Bohn et al., Sjostrand and co-workers[8,9] in Sweden developed a series of devices designed to decrease some of the hemodynamic consequences, such as decreases in cardiac output and metabolic acidosis, known to be associated with conventional mechanical ventilation. By decreasing ventilator tubing compliance, lowering the compressible volume of the ventilator, and using a specialized insufflation catheter, they could achieve rapid ventilator rates without appreciable loss of gas pressure within the system. Using rapid rates, they attained adequate alveolar ventilation at lower maximal and lower mean airway pressures than those required with conventional ventilators. These ventilators, through HFPPV, provided adequate ventilation and oxygenation. The circulatory compromise frequently seen with conventional forms of assisted ventilation was avoided because less pressure was applied to the pulmonary vasculature.

III. RELATIONSHIP OF HFV TO NEONATAL HEMODYNAMICS

In few patients is the therapeutic potential of HFV as great as in the neonate. The neonatal pulmonary circulation and the pathophysiologic responses of the pulmonary circulation to a variety of stimuli are unique to this age group.

In utero, the fetus has pathways for blood flow that allow shunting of blood from the gasless lungs to the systemic circulation, where it can reach the placenta for gaseous exchange. These fetal pathways, first described by Galen in the second century A.D., are the ductus arteriosus, ductus venosus, and the foramen ovale.[10] In most cases, the ductus arteriosus and ductus venosus remain anatomically patent for days to weeks after birth; the foramen ovale may remain patent until adulthood. Flow follows these pathways, depending on the difference between pulmonary and systemic vascular resistances. If the channels remain patent, the newborn may revert to a fetal pattern of cardiopulmonary blood flow in the extrauterine environment under circumstances of increased pulmonary vascular resistance or decreased systemic vascular resistance. If this happens, unsaturated blood flows from right to left at the atrial level via the foramen ovale, and from right to left at the ductus arteriosus. The consequence of both of these derangements in flow is significant systemic oxygen desaturation and cyanosis. This clinical syndrome of persistent fetal circulation, also called persistent pulmonary hypertension of the newborn, may lead to significant morbidity or death.

To understand this unique relationship between the pulmonary circulation and the systemic circulation in the neonate, one needs to consider the changes that occur in the fetal lung and cardiopulmonary circulation at birth. Dawes[11] was the first to describe in detail changes in fetal circulation at birth (Figure 1). With the expansion of the lungs and the establishment of an air-alveolar interface, there is a sudden drop in pulmonary vascular resistance.[12] As a result, pulmonary blood flow increases as well as venous return to the left atrium. The increase in left atrial return and in left atrial pressure causes the foramen ovale to functionally close, reducing or eliminating any right-to-left atrial shunting. Along with the drop in pulmonary vascular resistance, the systemic vascular resistance rises, due primarily to removal of the fetus from the placenta. Systemic vascular resistance then exceeds pulmonary vascular resistance and ductal flow reverses, now going let to right. Synchronization of the drop in pulmonary vascular resistance and the reduction in caliber of the ductus is a prerequisite for prevention of left ventricular failure.[13] In normal term infants, very little, if any, shunt is detectable 20 hr after birth, indicating that the ductus is functionally closed. Persistent patency of the ductus arteriosus is a common problem in the premature neonate, however, and presents unique problems when mechanical ventilatory support is required — a point to be discussed later in this chapter.

The progressive development of the pulmonary vascular bed and the increase in pulmonary vascular smooth muscle in the later stages of gestation have been described in both animals and humans.[14,15] This arteriolar smooth muscle regresses to approximately one half between birth and 2 to 3 weeks of postnatal age. Further, Rudolph and Yuan have demonstrated a significant vasoconstrictive response in the calf fetus and neonate to hypoxemia, which is enhanced by the coexistence of acidosis (Figure 2).[16] During fetal life, pulmonary vasoconstriction and reduced pulmonary blood flow is of little consequence. However, once exposed to the extrauterine environment, the neonate may develop acidosis and worsening pulmonary vascular resistance as a result of the pulmonary vasoconstriction. In addition, West[17] has shown that lung volume and

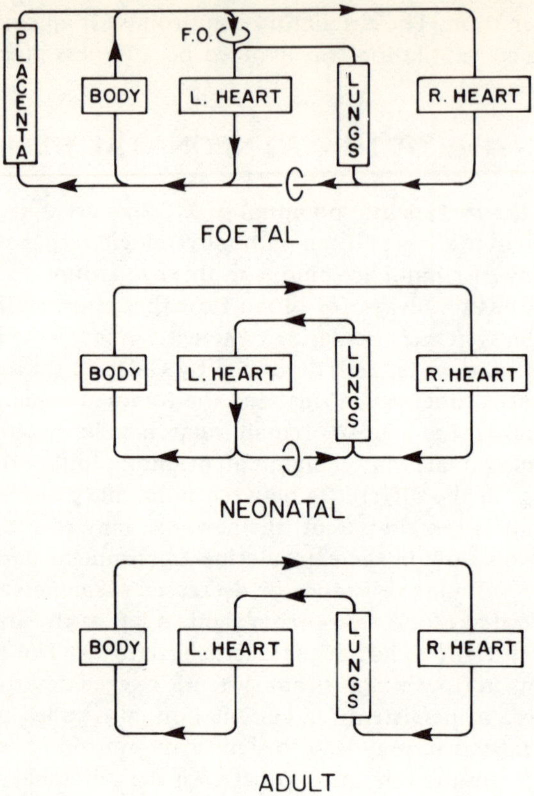

FIGURE 1. Dawes (1954) classic illustration of the postnatal changes in the circulation. (From Dawes, G. S., *Foetal and Neonatal Physiology. A Comparative Study of the Changes at Birth,* Year Book Publishers, Chicago, 1968. With permission.)

pressure exerted on the intra-alveolar resistance vessels may increase pulmonary vascular resistance to fetal levels and produce a resumption of fetal shunting. By increasing intrathoracic pressure, mechanical positive pressure ventilation will serve only to further heighten the pulmonary vascular resistance in these infants. Use of a ventilation technique that causes less mechanical distention of the alveoli while maintaining adequate ventilation would be important in decreasing detrimental effects of positive pressure ventilation.

IV. PRODUCTION OF VASOACTIVE SUBSTANCES

In addition to the influence of mechanical events associated with birth, the newborn must adjust biochemically to its new environment. Several prostaglandins are released with ventilation of a newborn lung; they are thought to be important in the overall regulation of pulmonary blood flow.[18] In addition to the involvement of prostaglandins in blood flow regulation, the regulation of regional blood flow in a variety of organs is believed to result from a complex balance between the prostaglandins, prostacyclin, and thromboxane A_2.

Shear stress generated by lung inflation using mechanical ventilation has been shown to stimulate the release of prostacyclin (PGI_2) from the pulmonary vasculature.[18] PGI_2 is a potent pulmonary vasodilator, known to attenuate the pulmonary vasoconstrictor

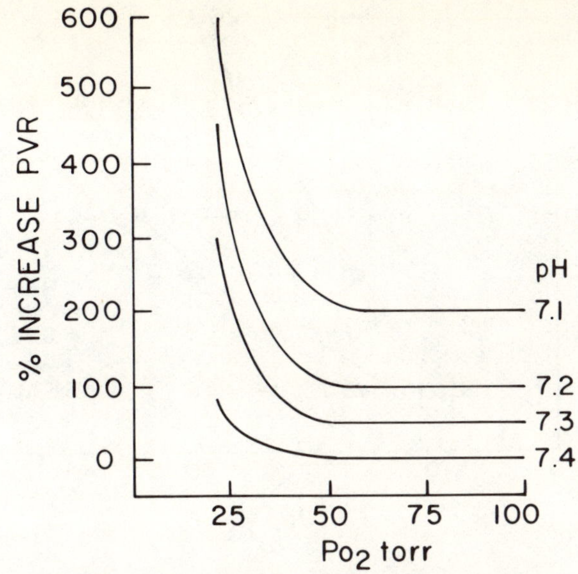

FIGURE 2. The effects of changes in PO_2, in pH alone and in both, on the pulmonary vascular resistance as derived from studies in newborn calves. (From Rudolph, A. M., *Congenital Diseases of the Heart,* Copyright 1974 by Year Book Medical Publishers Inc., Chicago. With permission.)

response to hypoxia. It probably plays an important role in modulating pulmonary vascular tone.[19,20] Wetzel et al.[21] studied the effect of the prostaglandin synthesis inhibitor, indomethacin, on the isolated, perfused lungs of sheep; one group was pretreated with indomethacin and a control group was untreated. They studied the response of the pulmonary vasculature by generating pressure-flow curves at various levels of oxygen tension in addition to determining the level of the prostacyclin metabolite (6-keto-prostaglandin $F_1\alpha$). The lungs were alternately ventilated with conventional ventilation and with HFV using a motor-driven flow interruptor at 1200 breaths per minute and a tidal volume less than 2 $m\ell/kg$. During hypoxia (PaO_2 = 30 torr), the pressure-flow relationship was significantly attenuated during HFV, although no differences between conventional ventilation and HFV occurred (Figure 3). The production of 6-keto-prostaglandin $F_1\alpha$ was higher in hypoxic sheep during HFV than during conventional ventilation. Indomethacin pretreatment abolished this effect. These studies suggest that more of the pulmonary vasodilator prostacyclin is produced with HFV than with conventional ventilation and that the increased flow per pressure unit during HFV may be related to the increased production of this compound. The data of Wetzel and colleagues suggest that factors other than lower distending pressures associated with the use of HFV may improve pulmonary blood flow in cases where pulmonary vascular resistance is high.

V. PERSISTENT FETAL CIRCULATION AND PULMONARY HYPERTENSION

Persistent fetal circulation presents a marked challenge to the health professionals who care for extremely sick infants with this problem. Many kinds of treatment have been investigated. These include manipulation of the pulmonary circulation by pharmacologic means as well as hyperventilation by mechanical ventilation. Fox and co-

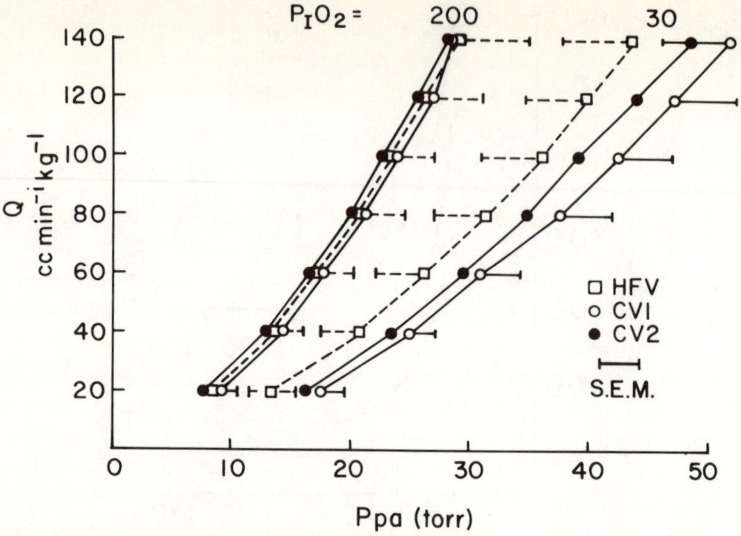

FIGURE 3. Pulmonary artery flow (Q) vs. pulmonary artery pressure (P_{pa}) at PIO_2 = 200 torr and 30 torr for both conventional (CV) and HVC. CV_1 and CV_2 are the first (pre HFV) and second (post HFV) runs respectively for CV. The points represent means ± SEM for five animals. At PIO_2 = 20 torr, there is no difference between the curves. At PIO_2 = 30 torr the HFV curve is significantly attenuated from both the CV_1 and CV_2 curves. (From Wetzel, R. C., et al., Int. Symp. High Frequency Ventilation, New York, 1983. With permission.)

workers[22] found that hypoxic infants with pulmonary hypertension responded to hyperventilation at rates that would reduce $PaCO_2$ to the 15 to 25 torr range, yielding a pH above 7.6. At these levels, pulmonary artery pressures and pulmonary vascular resistance fell below systemic levels, with a subsequent rise in pulmonary blood flow and systemic oxygenation. Unfortunately high peak inspiratory pressures and fast ventilation rates can result in high MAP that can be transmitted to the resistance vessels, leading to elevated pulmonary vascular resistance, and to resumption of fetal shunting. MAP lower than those created by conventional ventilation are possible with HFV, which seems to hold theoretical promise for lowering pulmonary vascular resistance in infants with persistent fetal circulation.

Patients with diseases in which high pulmonary artery pressures are a major component of the pathophysiology have been treated with HFV. Systematic trials still remain to be done. Certain patients with pulmonary hypertension also have pulmonary hypoplasia. Probably the most frustrating example of this group of diseases is congenital diaphragmatic hernia. In most neonatal centers the mortality from this entity is in excess of 50%.[23,24] Various modes of HFV have been tried for these infants, the rationale being to minimize the pressures exerted on their underdeveloped lung with coexisting compromised pulmonary vasculature. The outcome has been less promising than originally anticipated;[25,26] most of the severely affected infants die. However, most of the infants treated with HFV demonstrate an increase in CO_2 elimination on HFV compared to those who received conventional ventilation. Apparently, pulmonary hypoplasia and pulmonary arteriolar muscular hypertrophy in these infants were the critical factors leading to death. Certainly more systematic investigations are needed in this group of infants to determine whether or not HFV is efficacious in theirs treatment. A clinical scoring system such as that reported by Bohn et al.[27] for use in predict the eventual outcome would be useful in such studies, to determine which patients would die if only conventional treatments were used. An improvement in survival in such a group of patients would offer supportive evidence for the superiority of alternative modes of treatment such as HFV or Extra Corporeal Membrane Oxygenation.

VI. PREMATURE INFANTS WITH PATENT DUCTUS ARTERIOSUS

In premature infants in whom ductal patency may present the problem of left-to-right shunting with subsequent ventricular failure, Ackerman et al.[28] and Yoder et al.[29] have shown that HFV with low airway pressure may cause hypoxemia, hypercarbia, and severe diffuse atelectasis. They postulated that with HFV, lower alveolar pressures permitted a greater flow left to right through the ductus arteriosus. In addition, pulmonary production of vasodilating substances stimulated by ventilation, may encourage ductal patency. This is a potential detriment for this group of infants since it may worsen their respiratory compromise on the basis of cardiac failure. More studies are needed to develop appropriate ventilatory strategies that will obviate this HFV-generated ductal patency. Perhaps combinations of HFV superimposed with PEEP and intermittent conventional ventilator breaths will be the solution to this problem.

VII. HEMODYNAMIC EFFECTS OF CONVENTIONAL VENTILATION

The hemodynamic effects of positive pressure ventilation have been appreciated for more than 50 years.[30,31] Much of this early work remains valid to this day. Cournand et al.[32] were among the first to recognize that it was not simply positive intrathoracic pressure that affected hemodynamic change. Rather, it was the pattern of pressure during continuous positive pressure ventilation (CPPV) that played an important role. They found that cardiac output was diminished significantly with the onset of mechanical ventilation, but with a rapid inspiration and long expiratory times (inspiratory:expiratory ratios $\geq$ 1:2) this effect on cardiac output was minimal.

Subsequent studies[33-40] have confirmed and expanded upon the early work. Consistent findings have been that CPPV causes a decrease in venous return to the right side of the heart, an increase in pulmonary vascular resistance, and a decrease in stroke volume and cardiac output. Morgan et al.[36] found that with a rise in intrathoracic pressure, vena caval flow declined, leading to lowered pulmonary flow and ultimately lowered cardiac output. In attempts to simplify understanding of the effect of CPPV, some have described it as "a series of short, repeated Valsalva maneuvers".[41]

Logically, the next step would be to find a common denominator, such as mean intrathoracic pressure, which could be measured or estimated to explain these hemodynamic changes. As a major contributor to intrathoracic pressure, the amount of PEEP used during CPPV would seem to be important when one considers the hemodynamic effect that ventilation may have. Many workers have have studied the cardiovascular effects of PEEP[39,42-46] In general, the effect of PEEP, elevated pulmonary vascular resistance and a lowered cardiac output is proportional to the amount of end-expiratory pressure applied. However, this is more complex than a simple cause-and-effect relationship. Attempts to mimic the effect of PEEP by surgically[34] or mechanically[46] creating resistance to pulmonary blood flow (i.e., artificially increasing pulmonary vascular resistance) have shown that cardiac output does not necessarily decline; therefore other factors (perhaps neuronal or humoral) are involved. However, Fuhrman and co-workers,[47] using unilateral changes in PEEP in one lung and measurement of individual lung blood flows, recently reported that with increases in unilateral PEEP, ipsilateral but not contralateral pulmonary blood flow was affected. The major effect was on the ipsilateral lung, and little or no indirect effect was found on the contralateral lung. Therefore the major effect of PEEP would appear to be *direct*.

These same authors also found that the effect of PEEP on the pulmonary vasculature was not determined by static pressure alone.[48] They found that a unilateral application of a continuous positive airway pressure (CPAP) decreased pulmonary blood flow to the lung in which it was applied. But, a pulsatile airway pressure (CPPV) had a much larger effect on blood flow than CPAP alone; CPPV with 10 cm H_2O PEEP decreased blood flow as much as CPAP with 25 cm H_2O.

Hemodynamic responses to ventilation also occur in extrathoracic structures. An intracranial pressure increase is mediated by a rise in superior vena cava pressure and a fall in cerebral venous outflow.[49] Neonates are particularly sensitive to intrathoracic pressure changes that result in elevations of venous pressure being transmitted to cerebral vessels.[50] Because of the fragility of certain neonatal cerebral vessels, when acute intrathoracic pressure changes occur (as in pneumothorax) intracranial hemorrhage may result.[51] Hemodynamic changes in other major organ systems are less well studied. Portal and hepatic flow is decreased with CPPV out of proportion to changes in cardiac output.[52,53] Splanchnic and renal blood flow are also affected[54] and urine output may diminish.[39]

VIII. HEMODYNAMIC EFFECTS OF HFV

HFV by virtue of its ability to maintain adequate ventilation with small tidal volume, avoids creating the large intrathoracic pressure swings seen with conventional ventilation. However, HFV has an overall effect on hemodynamic function similar to that found with conventional ventilation. Early studies with HFOV showed that adequate ventilation could be maintained while cardiac output remained similar to that in conventional ventilation.[6,7] Initial studies with HFJV showed similar results:[55,56] the cardiac output remained similar to that seen with conventional ventilation. HFV does cause amplitude modulation at specific "beat frequencies" in several cardiovascular measurements, with pulmonary artery pressure displaying the most prominent pattern.[57] The physiologic significance of these modulations is not clear, as no important changes in cardiovascular function are associated with them.

There may be some hemodynamic benefit or improvement from HFV. Carlon et al.[58] studied several patients for whom conventional ventilation had failed and who were given a trial of jet ventilation; even though cardiac output itself was unchanged, the patients could be weaned from cardiotonic agents. A recent animal study[59] has shown improved hemodynamic function resulting from jet ventilation compared to conventional ventilation. Cardiac output was consistently higher with jet ventilation, even at the same MAP as CPPV.

Attempts to improve cardiac output by synchronizing HFJV cycles with heart rate have been interesting, but not highly successful. Carlon et al.[60,61] reported increased cardiac output and ejection fraction with synchronization; however, results were inconsistent and unpredictable.

Comprehensive studies in infants have been lacking. The most complete measurement of hemodynamic parameters has been done by Vincent et al.,[62] who measured hemodynamic response to short term HFV in infants who had just undergone cardiac surgery. No significant changes in cardiac output were seen, although pulmonary artery pressure and pulmonary vascular resistance increased, possibly secondary to airtrapping or inadvertent PEEP.[63] HFV is known to cause inadvertent PEEP,[64] which is also an unmeasurable hazard of using conventional ventilators at high frequencies.[65] Although these are theoretical concerns,[66] limited clinical use of HFV has not confirmed them. In fact one may argue that inadvertent PEEP may be an integral part of the ventilation in abnormal or diseases lungs.[67]

The hemodynamic effect of HFV on extrathoracic structures has been studied most closely in the brain. HFV does not alter cerebral blood flow if normocarbia is maintained.[68] HFV has been found to decrease fluctuations in intracranial pressure normally seen with mechanical ventilation,[69,70] and it diminishes surface movement of the brain,[71] which may make it an ideal ventilation technique for neurosurgical procedures.

Renal response to HFV has not been well studied. One clinical study[72] did include the measurement of plasma renin activity with altered levels of PEEP during HFJV. Zero PEEP maintained normal plasma renin activity and renal function, while the addition of PEEP raised renin activity and lowered renal function.

Little information is available regarding hemodynamic changes in other organ systems such as liver, gut, and endocrine glands. Gioia et al.[73] evaluated regional blood flow by using radiolabeled microspheres during CPPV and HFV. They found that HFV caused no circulatory changes when compared to CPPV; regional blood flows during HFV and CPPV were similar in all organs studied, including liver, adrenal glands, pancreas, kidney (medulla and cortex), jejunum, skeletal muscle, and central nervous system. The majority of information available in the literature refers to hemodynamic changes in response to *hyperventilation* (which implies a decrease in $PaCO_2$ and increase in pH)[74,75] rather than HFV per se.

As alluded to previously, the hemodynamic effects of ventilation on extrathoracic structures appear to be complex. Apnea is known to occur with HFV[6,7] and many receptors and reflex arcs are implicated.[76-78] It is not clear at this time how these neuronal responses alter hemodynamic effects, but certainly the ability to alter and modify central nervous system functions (e.g., respiratory drive) has significant implications for the cardiovascular system. Also complicating the indirect effects are humoral factors: pulmonary-produced vasoactive substances such as prostaglandins,[79] whose local hemodynamic effects are well appreciated, but as yet of only theoretical importance in altering the hemodynamics of other organs.

The evaluation of hemodynamic response to mechanical ventilation is a complex undertaking for several reasons:

1. The response is the result of direct pressure effects interacting dynamically with indirect neuronally and humorally mediated forces.
2. Hemodynamic effects may already by overwhelmingly altered for other reasons, such as shock, cardiac failure, or hypovolemia.
3. The patient's underlying disease and clinical status will alter or modify effects; for example, stiff noncompliant lungs will not transmit pressures effectively, acid/base status will alter vascular reactivity, and the use of sedation or paralysis will greatly change muscle tone and modify neurologically mediated reflexes.

Just as a physician considers the risks and benefits of traditional therapies, so should the risks and benefits of HFV be considered. The clinician should remain cognizant of the potential for direct, as well as indirect, effects of HFV when he elects to use it, realizing that knowledge about the hemodynamic effects is critical, but limited.

REFERENCES

1. Henderson, Y., Chilligsworth, F. D., and Whitney, J. L., The respiratory dead spaces, *Am. J. Physiol.*, 338, 1, 1915.
2. Lunkenheimer, P. P., Frank, I., Ising, H., Keller, H., and Dickhut, H. H., Intrapulmoner Gaswechsel unter simulierter Apnoe durch transtrachealen periodischen intrathorakulen Druckwechsel, *Anesthetist*, 22, 232, 1973.

3. Lunkenheimer, P. P., Ising, H., Frank, I., Scharsich, M., Welham, K., and Dittrich, H., Enhancement of CO_2-elimination by intrapulmonary high frequency pressure alternation during "Apnoeic Oxygenation", *Adv. Exp. Med. Biol.*, 94, 599, 1977.
4. Lunkenheimer, P. P., Rafflenbeul, W., Keller, H., Frank, I., Dickhut, H. H., and Fuhrmann, C., Application of transtracheal pressure oscillations as modification of "Diffusion Respiration", *Br. J. Anaesthesiol.*, 44, 627, 1972.
5. Fukuchi, Y., Roussos, C. S., Macklem, P. T., and Engel, L. A., Convection, diffusion and cardiogenic mixing of inspired gas in the lung: an experimental approach, *Respir. Physiol.*, 26, 77, 1976.
6. Butler, W. J., Bohn, D. J., Miyasaka, K., Bryan, A. C., and Froese, A. B., Ventilation in humans by high frequency oscillation, *Anesth. Analg.*, 59, 577, 1980.
7. Bohn, D., Miyasaka, B. E., Marchak, W. K., Thompson, A. B., Froese, A. B., and Bryan, A. C., Ventilation by high frequency oscillation, *J. Appl. Physiol.*, 48, 710, 1980.
8. Sjostrand, U., Review of the physiological rationale for and development of high-frequency positive-pressure ventilation — HFPPV, *Acta Anaesthesiol. Scand.*, Suppl. 64, 7, 1977.
9. Sjostrand, U., High-frequency positive pressure ventilation (HFPPV): a review, *Crit. Care. Med.*, 8, 345, 1980.
10. Rashkine, W. J., A brief historical perspective, *Pediatr. Cardiol.*, 1, 62, 1979/80.
11. Dawes, G. S., *Foetal and Neonatal Physiology. A Comparative Study of the Changes at Birth*, Year Book, Chicago, 1968.
12. Cassin, S., Dawes, G. S., Mott, J. C., et al., Changes in the heart and lungs at birth, in *Cold Springs Harbor Symp. Quantitative Biol.*, Vol. 14, New York, 1954.
13. Wallgren, G., Den centrala cirkulationshostallningen vid fodelsen, *Lakartidningen*, 74, 1708, 1977.
14. Civin, W. W. and Edwards, J. E., Postnatal structural changes in the intrapulmonary arteries and arterioles, *AMA Arch. Pathol.*, 51, 192, 1951.
15. Naeye, R. L., Arterial changes during the perinatal period, *Arch. Pathol.*, 71, 121, 1961.
16. Rudolph, A. M. and Heymann, M. A., Circulatory changes with growth in the fetal lamb, *Circ. Res.*, 26, 298, 1970.
17. West, J. B., *Ventilation/Blood Flow and Gas Exchange*, Blackwell Scientific, Oxford, 1965.
18. Korbut, R., Boyd, J., and Eling, T., Respiratory movements alter the generation of prostacyclin and thromboxane A_2 in isolated rat lungs: the influence of arachidonic acid-pathway inhibitors on the ratio between pulmonary prostacylcin and thromboxane A_2, *Prostaglandins*, 21, 491, 1981.
19. Gregory, T. J., Newell, J. C., Hakim, T. S., Levitzky, M. G., and Sedansk, N., Attenuation of hypoxic pulmonary vaxoconstriction by pulsatile flow in dog lungs, *J. Appl. Physiol.*, 53, 1583, 1982.
20. Gerber, J. G., Voelkel, N., Nies, A. S., McMurty, I. F., and Reeves, J. T., Moderation of hypoxic vasoconstriction by infused arachidonic acid: role of PGI_2, *J. Appl. Physiol.*, 49, 107, 1980.
21. Wetzel, R. C., Gordon, J. B., Gregory, T. J., and Gioia, F. R., High frequency ventilation attenuates the pulmonary vascular response to hypoxia, in Int. Symp. High Frequency Ventilation, New York, Nov. 18 to 20, 1983. 77.
22. Fox, W. W. and Duara, S., Persistent pulmonary hypertension of the neonate: diagnosis and clinical management, *J. Pediatr.*, 103, 505, 1983.
23. Mishlaney, H. G., Konsouke, N., and Wooley, M. M., Congenital diaphragmatic hernia: eleven years experience, *Arch. Surg.*, 114, 1118, 1979.
24. Ruff, S. J., Campbell, J. R., Harrison, M. R., et al., Pediatric diaphragmatic hernia: an eleven year experience, *Am. J. Surg.*, 139, 641, 1980.
25. Neu, J., Hamilton, L., Linehan, J., et al., Long term high-frequency jet ventilation in neonates, *Crit. Care Med.*, 12, 833, 1984.
26. Bohn, D. J., Personal communication.
27. Bohn, D. J., James, I., Filler, R. M., Ein, S. H., Wesson, D. E., Shandling, B., Stephens, C., and Barker, G. A., The relationship between $PaCO_2$ and ventilation parameters in predicting survival in congenital diaphragmatic hernia, *J. Pediatr. Surg.*, 19, 666, 1984.
28. Ackerman, N. B., Kuel, T. J., et al., Cardiovascular interactions with high frequency ventilation: preliminary observations in premature baboons with hyaline membrane disease, *Crit. Care Med.*, 12, 338, 1984.
29. Yoder, B. A., Ackerman, N. B., et al., The effect of mechanical ventilation on left to right ductal shunting in immature baboons, *Crit. Care Med.*, 12, 376, 1984.
30. Huggett, A. St. G., Studies on the respiration and circulation of the cat, *J. Physiol.*, 59, 373, 1924.
31. Humphrey, G. H., Moore, R. L., Maier, H. C., et al., Studies of the cardiac output of anesthetized dogs during continuous and intermittent inflation of the lungs, *J. Thorac. Surg.*, 7, 438, 1938.
32. Cournand, A., Motley, H. L., Werko, L., and Richards, D. W., Physiological studies of the effects of intermittent positive pressure breathing on cardiac output in man, *Am. J. Physiol.*, 152, 162, 1938.
33. Briscoe, W. A., Forster, R. E., and Comroe, J. H., Alveolar ventilation at very low tidal volumes, *J. Appl. Physiol.*, 7, 27, 1954.

34. Braunwald, E., Binion, J. T., Morgan, W. L., Jr., and Sarnoff, S. J., Alteration in central blood volume and cardiac output induced by positive pressure breathing and counteracted by metaraminol (Aramine), *Circ. Res.*, 5, 670, 1957.
35. Watson, W. E., Observations on physiological deadspace during intermittent positive pressure respiration, *Br. J. Anaesth.*, 34, 502, 1962.
36. Morgan, B. C., Martin, W. E., Hornbein, T. F., Crawford, E. W., and Guntheroth, W. G., Hemodynamic effects of intermittent positive pressure respiration, *Anesthesiology*, 27, 584, 1966.
37. Prys-Roberts, C., Kelman, G. R., and Greenbaum, R., The influence of circulatory factors on arterial oxygenation in man, *Anesthesia*, 22, 257, 1967.
38. Ashbaugh, D. G., Effect of ventilatory methods and patterns on physiologic shunt, *Surgery*, 68, 99, 1970.
39. Qvist, J., Pontoppidan, H., Wilson, R. S., Lowenstein, E., and Laver, M. B., Hemodynamic responses to mechanical ventilation with PEEP: the effect of hypervolemia, *Anesthesiology*, 42, 45, 1975.
40. Cassidy, S. S., Eschenbacher, W. L., Robertson, C. H., Jr., Nixon, J. V., Blomquist, G., and Johnson, R. L., Jr., Cardiovascular effects of positive pressure ventilation in normal subjects, *J. Appl. Physiol.*, 47, 453, 1979.
41. Conway, C. M., Haemodynamic effects of pulmonary ventilation, *Br. J. Anaesth.*, 47, 761, 1975.
42. Hobelmann, C. F., Jr., Smith, D. E., Virgilio, R. W., Shapiro, A. R., and Peters, R. M., Hemodynamic alterations with positive end-expiratory pressure: the contribution of the pulmonary vasculature, *J. Trauma*, 15, 951, 1975.
43. Powers, S. R. and Manual, R., Physiologic consequences of positive end-expiratory ventilation, *Ann. Surg.*, 178, 265, 1973.
44. MacConnell, K. F., Lefemine, A. A., Moon, H. S., Donovan, D. J., and Johnston, R. P., Comparative hemodynamic consequences of inflation hold, PEEP and interrupted PEEP, *Ann. Thorac. Surg.*, 19, 552, 1975.
45. Jardin, F., Farcot, J. C., Borsanti, L., Curien, N., Margeuraz, B., and Bourdarias, J. P., Influence of positive end-expiratory pressure on left ventricular performance, *N. Engl. J. Med.*, 304, 387, 1981.
46. Liebman, P. R., Patten, M. T., Mammy, J., Shepro, D., and Hechtman, H. B., The mechanism of depressed cardiac output on positive end-expiratory pressure (PEEP), *Surgery*, 83, 594, 1978.
47. Fuhrman, B. P., Everitt, J., and Lock, J. E., Cardiopulmonary effects of unilateral airway pressure changes in intact infant lambs, *J. Appl. Physiol.*, 56, 1439, 1984.
48. Furhman, B. P., Kulik, T. J., Smith-Wright, D. L., Spotts, B. A., and Lock, J. E., A greater effect of pulsatile than of static airway pressure on the pulmonary vasculature, *Crit. Care Med.*, 11 (Abstr.), 215, 1983.
49. Lace, J. M., Huseby, J. S., Kird, W., et al., Mechanism by which positive end-expiratory pressure increases cerebrospinal fluid pressure in dogs, *J. Appl. Physiol.*, 52, 231, 1982.
50. De Lemos, R. A. and Tomasovic, J. T., Effects of positive pressure ventilation on cerebral blood flow in the newborn infant, *Clin. Perinatol.*, 5, 395, 1978.
51. Hill, A., Perlamn, J. M., and Volpe, J. J., Relationship of pneumothorax to occurance of intraventricular hemorrhage in the premature newborn, *Pediatrics*, 69, 144, 1982.
52. Bonnet, F., Richard, C., Glaser, P., et al., Changes in hepatic flow induced by continuous positive pressure ventilation in critically ill patients, *Crit. Care Med.*, 10, 703, 1982.
53. Johnson, E. E. and Hedley-Whyte, J., Continuous positive pressure ventilation and portal flow in dogs with pulmonary edema, *J. Appl. Physiol.*, 33, 385, 1972.
54. Hedley-Whyte, J., Burgess, G. E., Feeley, T. N., et al., Effect of pattern of ventilation on heaptic renal and splanchnic function, in *Applied Physiology of Respiratory Care*, Little, Brown, Boston, 1976, 27.
55. Schuster, D. P., Klain, M., and Snyder, J. V., Comparison of high frequency jet ventilation to conventional ventilation during severe acute respiratory failure in humans, *Crit. Care Med.*, 10, 625, 1982.
56. Hoff, B. H., Smith, R. B., Bunegin, L., and Cherry, B., High frequency ventilation in dogs with open chests, *Crit. Care Med.*, 10, 517, 1982.
57. Pinchak, A. C., Hagen, J. F., Hancock, D. E., and Kovijanic, C., Beat frequencies in high-frequency positive-pressure ventilation, *Crit. Care Med.*, 12, 729, 1984.
58. Carlon, G. C., Kahn, R. C., Howland, W. S., Ray, C., and Turnbull, A. D., Clinical experience with high frequency jet ventilation, *Crit. Care Med.*, 9, 1, 1981.
59. Chiaranda, M., Rubini, A., Fiore, G., Giron, G., and Carlon, G. C., Hemodynamic effects of continuous positive-pressure ventilation and high frequency jet ventilation with positive end-expiratory pressure in normal dogs, *Crit. Care Med.*, 12, 750, 1984.
60. Carlon, G., Pierri, M. K., Groeger, J., et al., Cardiac counterpulsation using high frequency jet ventilation, *Crit. Care Med.*, 11 (Abstr.), 244, 1983.

61. Carlon, G. C., Ray, C., Pierri, M. K., Groeger, J., and Howland, W. S., High-frequency jet ventilation: theoretical considerations and clinical observations, *Chest,* 81, 350, 1982.
62. Vincent, R. N., Stark, A. R., Lang, P., Close, R. H., et al., Hemodynamic response to high-frequency ventilation in infants following cardiac surgery, *Pediatrics,* 73, 426, 1984.
63. Brady, J. P., *Neonatal Pulmonary Care,* Thibeault, D. W. and Gregory, G. A., Eds., Menlo Park, Calif., 1979, 310.
64. Beamer, W. C., Prough, D. S., Royster, R. L., Johnston, W. E., and Johnson, J. C., High-frequency jet ventilation produces auto-PEEP, *Crit. Care Med.,* 12, 734, 1984.
65. Hagen, E. A., Bucciarelli, R. L., and Jaeger, M. J., "Inadvertent PEEP" with the use of a conventional ventilator is undetected by a proximal airway pressure monitor, *Pediatr. Res.,* 18 (Abstr.), 393A, 1984.
66. Weigel, J., The infant lung: a case against high respiratory ratios in controlled neonatal ventilation, *Resp. Ther.,* 3, 57, 1973.
67. Cartwright, D. W., Willis, M. M., and Gregory, G. A., Functional residual capacity and lung mechanics at different levels of mechanical ventilation, *Crit. Care Med.,* 12, 44, 1984.
68. Toutant, S. M., Todd, M. M., Drummond, J. C., and Shapiro, H. M., Cerebral blood flow during high frequency ventilation in cats, *Crit. Care Med.,* 11, 712, 1983.
69. Babinski, M. F., Albin, M., and Smith, R. B., Effect of high frequency ventilation in ICP, *Crit. Care Med.,* 9, 159, 1981.
70. Raju, T. N. K., Braverman, B., Nadkarny, U., Kim, W. K., and Vidyasager, D., Intracranial pressure and cardiac output remain stable during high frequency oscillation, *Crit. Care Med.,* 11, 856, 1983.
71. Todd, M. M., Toutant, S. M., and Shapiro, H. M., The effects of high-frequency ventilation on intracranial pressure and brain surface movement in cats, *Anesthesiology,* 54, 496, 1981.
72. Marquez, J., Guntupalli, K., Sladen, A., and Klain, M., Renal function and renin secretion during high frequency jet ventilation at varying levels of airway pressure, *Crit. Care Med.,* 11, 930, 1983.
73. Gioia, F. R., Harris, A. P., Hamburger, C., Parker, S. D., Traystman, R. J., and Roger, M. C., Peripheral circulatory changes with high frequency ventilation, *Anesthesiology,* 55, A357, 1981.
74. Sola, A., Spitzer, A. R., Morin, F. C., Schlueter, M. A., and Phibbs, R. H., Effects of arterial carbon dioxide tension on the newborn lamb's cardiovascular responses to rapid hemorrhage, *Pediatr. Res.,* 17, 70, 1983.
75. Johnson, E. E., Splanchnic hemodynamic response to passive hyperventilation, *J. Appl. Physiol.,* 38, 156, 1975.
76. England, S. J., Onayemi, A., and Bryan, A. C., Neuromuscular blockade enhances phrenic nerve activity during high-frequency ventilation, *J. Appl. Physiol.,* 56, 31, 1984.
77. Thompson, W. K., Marchak, B. E., Bryan, A. C., and Froese, A. B., Vagotomy reverses apnea induced by high-frequency oscillatory ventilation, *J. Appl. Physiol.,* 51, 1484, 1981.
78. Banzett, R., Lehr, J., and Geffroy, B., High-frequency ventilation lengthens expiration in the anesthetized dog, *J. Appl. Physiol.,* 55, 329, 1983.
79. Leffler, C. W., Hessler, J. R., and Terragno, N. A., Ventilation induced release of prostaglandin-like material from fetal lungs, *Am. J. Physiol.,* 238, H282, 1980.

Chapter 7

HIGH-FREQUENCY VENTILATION IN PEDIATRICS AND NEONATOLOGY

D. J. Bohn, M. Tamura, and A. C. Bryan

TABLE OF CONTENTS

I. INTRODUCTION

Throughout the past two decades, the use of mechanical ventilation has significantly lowered the mortality of neonates from a variety of newborn respiratory diseases: e.g., infant respiratory distress syndrome (IRDS), meconium aspiration, congenital diaphragmatic hernia, and persistent fetal circulation. In the 1970s the introduction of PEEP and CPAP was shown to be beneficial in patients with respiratory failure whose lung compliance was reduced due to either primary or secondary surfactant deficiency. However, with advances in neonatal intensive care, the increasing use of ventilation for premature and low birth weight infants with immature lungs has resulted in the development of more chronic lung disease; this has been variously ascribed to the effects of positive pressure, inspired oxygen level, and the duration of ventilation.

The respirators originally used for ventilating infants were machines in which volumes and frequencies had been designed for adult use. They proved less than satisfactory when adapted to the pediatric patient. Not until the 1970s did specific "pediatric" ventilators become available, generally of the pressure-limited, time-cycled variety. They were designed with the concept that mechanical ventilation in small infants should slavishly imitate the rates and volumes seen with spontaneous respiration in normal neonates. While this theory may make good physiological sense for infants with normal lungs, it may be inappropriate for infants with severe interstitial or alveolar lung disease. At the same time, awareness was increasing that, for small infants with immature lungs, the respirator may be not only part of the solution but part of the problem. In lung disease associated with low pulmonary compliance, the high shearing forces necessary to open collapsed alveoli during both spontaneous and positive pressure ventilation may lead to chronic lung damage. Since Northway's original description of bronchopulmonary dysplasia secondary to IRDS,[1] the debate has continued regarding the relative contributions of pressure and oxygen in its etiology. While the precise cause may be debatable the problem remains real enough. The reported incidence is between 5 and 38%, depending on diagnostic criteria and study population.[2-4] The incidence will rise with the increased survival of low birth weight infants, approaching 40% in infants 1000 g.

More recently, the concern about pulmonary barotrauma in both mature and immature lungs of infants has translated into an attempt to reduce damage to the lung parencyma by reducing peak airway pressures while simultaneously increasing ventilator frequencies (1 to 2 Hz) to compensate for the decrease in minute volume.[5] While this technique has proved effective as a method of CO_2 elimination, whether it lessens barotrauma or improves oxygenation remains to be determined. With the success of techniques such as these, the logic of using conventional respirator rates and volumes in patients with parenchymal lung disease weakens, and the problems of CO_2 elimination and oxygenation need to be addressed separately. A more rational approach is to separate the causes of respiratory failure into "pump" failure, indicating disease of respiratory muscles, central respiratory drive, or the thoracic cage, and "lung" failure, indicating disease of the airways, alveoli, or interstitial space.[6] The former is characterized by CO_2 retention and the latter by hypoxemia. "Pump" failure may be managed adequately with conventional ventilator techniques. However, "lung" failure represents a far more difficult management problem, with a greater potential for further damaging the diseased lung.

With the advent of HFV (> 2 Hz), the concept that net bulk flow is necessary for gas transport has been proved to be incorrect. Augmented gas diffusion, without major pressure changes in the airway, may be a far more efficient method of gas transport. There are good reasons then, why alternative ventilation strategies should be considered in infants whose immature lungs and reduced lung compliance present major problems in gas exchange.

II. RESPIRATORY FAILURE IN THE NEWBORN PERIOD

A. IRDS

Since the treatment of IRDS by positive pressure ventilation was first reported 25 years ago,[7] a wealth of experience has accumulated on the management of this and other causes of respiratory failure in the newborn. This and the advent of CPAP in 1971[8] have significantly lowered the mortality due to IRDS and other forms of interstitial and alveolar lung disease.

Of all the causes of neonatal respiratory failure, the most information is available on IRDS, in terms of both the pathological process and the effect of therapy on the diseased lung. Macroscopically, the lungs are of small volume, are airless, and have multiple areas of atelectasis. Diffuse hyaline membranes form at respiratory bronchiole, alveolar duct, and air saccule levels. Pulmonary edema develops in both interstitial and alveolar spaces.[9,10] The hyaline membranes themselves are the result of epithelial cell necrosis and protein deposition; they are seen only in live-born, usually premature infants, whether they are breathing spontaneously or are on mechanical ventilation.[11,12] Although it has been claimed that hyaline membranes in newborn humans do not form until after 2 hr of life, endothelial cell changes and edema formation occur within the first few hours of life.[13-15] In animal models (premature monkeys and rabbits), hyaline membrane formation has been shown to occur within 5 min of the onset of positive pressure ventilation.[16,17] Hyaline membrane formation has little to do with the etiology of IRDS and it is a nonspecific response of the lung to injury that occurs in both IRDS and adult respiratory distress syndrome (ARDS). In IRDS, surfactant deficiency results in increased alveolar surface tension, and the high transpulmonary distending pressures that produce hyaline membranes are equally likely to occur with either spontaneous or positive pressure ventilation. While in ARDS there is no primary surfactant abnormality, there may be qualitative and distributive abnormalities. Indeed, it is becoming increasingly evident that IRDS and ARDS are but two variants of acute lung injury and that the lung has a limited repertoire of responses to acute injury. The main responses are increasing endothelial premeability, epithelial cell damage, and edema formation. This results in proliferaton of type II cells and fibroblast infiltration leading to fibrosis, features common to all types of acute lung injury. One of the singular features of ARDS was thought to be neutrophil migration into the lung, but recent studies have shown that pulmonary neutrophil activity is also increased in IRDS.[18,19] Hyaline membranes are as likely to form in adults as in infants.[20-22] Earlier studies have suggested that the site of hyaline membrane formation differs between adult and infant varieties of the disease.[23-25] More recent evidence suggests that the site of formation at respiratory bronchiole and alveolar duct level is common to both diseases.

Although the typical pathological features of IRDS are well known, the relative contributions of disease and therapy to the lung injury are difficult to determine. Factors such as the transudation of plasma proteins,[26,27] ineffective pulmonary fibrinolytic activity,[19,20,22,28] and oxygen toxicity[19,20,22,28] have been at one time or other, held responsible for hyaline membrane formation, while positive pressure ventilation was ignored as a common factor in all instances. More recent studies have clearly implicated the high transpulmonary distending pressures associated with mechanical ventilation as being responsible for most of the pathological changes.[16,17,29,30] In an animal model (rabbits), both Nillson[16] and Schwieler and Robertson[29] have been able to produce hyaline membrane formation and bronchiolar epithelial damage after short periods of positive pressure ventilation. Schweiler and Robertson compared liquid ventilation to positive pressure ventilation in premature rabbits, and demonstrated definite lung damage with mechanical ventilation. They have argued that the air-liquid interface in the atelectatic lung of the infant with IRDS, is in the terminal conducting airways and that the primary site of damage is here, rather than in the alveoli. When applied to this interface the distending forces distort the bronchiole because the tissue elastic forces here cannot overcome the pressure required to advance the interface, towards the alveolus. This damages and eventually disrupts of the epithelial lining; the debris of these sloughing epithelial cells form hyaline membranes.

Interstitial edema formation is a typical feature of IRDS in both animal models and human studies. Bressack and Bland[32] have shown that alveolar hypoxia increases pulmonary lymph flow in newborn lambs without producing edema. They attributed this to an increase in pulmonary vascular hydrostatic pressure without a change in endothelial permeability. In contrast, the same protocol in mature sheep showed no change in pulmonary lymph flow with alveolar hypoxia, suggesting that the pulmonary microvascular circulation responds differently in the immature lung.[31-32] Hansen et al.[33] confirmed this in lambs, and also demonstrated that this increase in pulmonary lymph with no change in protein content was independent of changes in pleural pressure and $PaCO_2$ levels; it occurred during both spontaneous and positive pressure ventilation. No change was found in the wet weight:dry weight ratio of the lung tissue in these experiments. Although these experiments demonstrated no change in endothelial permeability, Egan et al.[34] demonstrated a change in epithelial permeability in lambs with hyaline membrane disease during the first few hours of ventilation. In this study, increased surfactant was released into the aveolar space during spontaneous breathing compared with mechanical ventilation; inspiratory positive pressure ventilation was associated with an increased flux of radiolabeled protein and increased lung water. Using a similar model, Jobe et al.[35] examined the permeability of the alveolar epithelium during mechanical ventilation; they demonstrated a bidirectional protein flux even before the development of hypoxemia. Furthermore, the instillation of natural surfactant into the lambs' lung's significantly reduced protein leakage, and resulted in increased PaO_2 and decreased peak inspiratory pressures (PIP) needed to support the animals. A direct relationship was found between the PIP and the degree of permeability, with increasing pressures causing increasing protein flux. These studies suggest that edema formation in IRDS may be due to changes in cardiodiopulmonary mechanics and damage to the normally impermeable epithelial membrane. This has been confirmed in infants; Jefferies et al.[36] showed a very rapid clearance of labeled aerosol from the lung in neonates with IRDS who inhaled ^{99m}Tc-DTPA, indicating increased permeability. Such damage could be made worse by positive pressure ventilation.

Kudoh[37] investigated the effect of positive pressure ventilation on the mature lung of dogs in oleic-acid-induced pulmonary edema, using each animal its own control. While lung was ventilated, the second was left merely inflated. The wet weight:dry weight ratio was consistently higher in the lung subjected to positive pressure ventilation.

The progression of IRDS to bronchopulmonary dysplasia has been well documented, although controversy exists over the relative contributions of oxygen and positive pressure. In his original description, Northway et al.[1] noted the similarity between the histological features of bronchopulmonary dysplasia and the vascular engorgement, edema, and epithelial necrosis that are characteristic of oxygen toxicity in all animal species.[38] This interpretation was supported by the experiments of De Lemos et al.[39] who were able to produce fatal lung edema in newborn lambs by ventilation with 100% oxygen for 2 to 4 days, but no damage by ventilation with air. Bronchopulmonary dysplasia has been reported in infants who have received only supplemental oxygen therapy without positive pressure ventilation.[40,41] Similar lesions typical of IRDS resulting in bronchopulmonary dysplasia and pulmonary fibrosis have been produced by exposure to high concentrations of inspired oxygen[42-47] leading to chronic lung disease. More convincing evidence, however, implicates the role of mechanical trauma in BPD.

Taghizadeh[48] and Reynolds[49] found a lower incidence of bronchopulmonary dysplasia in neonates when airway pressures during mechanical ventilation were below 35 cm H_2O. While other studies on hyaline membrane disease in humans are more equivocal, most tend to favor barotrauma as the main culprit in causing chronic lung disease in neonates.[50,51] While these issues may be disputable, there is little doubt that a combination of oxygen at high pressure and prolonged ventilation both contribute to damage to the immature lung.

III. THE LIMITATIONS OF CONVENTIONAL VENTILATION

A. Strategy for Hypoxic Lung Disease

The conventional solution to lung failure associated with parenchymal lung disease is to apply positive pressure to the lung in order to provide bulk flow of gases. While CO_2 transport to the exterior is more dependent on bulk transport because of its low diffusion gradient, oxygen transport is more diffusion-dependent; this characteristic is used to advantage in the apnoeic oxygenation technique. In diseases in which lung compliance is reduced, convective transport requires that the airway pressure exceed the opening pressure of collapsed segments enough for gas insufflation and CO_2 exchange to take place. However, because of the hysteresis phenomenon of the lung, terminal airway units close at a higher lung volume during expiration and alveolar collapse, and hypoxaemia ensues unless PEEP maintains the lung above opening pressure (around 15 cm H_2O).[52] Increasing the pressure levels above 15 cm H_2O may overcome this, but, added to the high inflation pressures already distorting terminal lung units, it will worsen pulmonary barotrauma. One strategy for dealing with this hypoxaemia is to prolong the inspiratory phase, thereby holding open terminal lung units for more of the respiratory cycle. This has been used to advantage in the treatment of IRDS by reversing the normal I:E ratio from 1:2 to 3:1 or 4:1 with a demonstrable improvement in oxygenation.[53] Boros[54] has shown the clear relationship between MAP and oxygenation in this disease. There is potential benefit, therefore, in devising an alternative strategy of ventilation that maintains lung inflation without the cyclical expansion and collapse of terminal lung units occurring with conventional ventilation.

IV. HFV IN ANIMAL MODELS OF HYALINE MEMBRANE DISEASE AND ACUTE LUNG INJURY

Since its inception, HFV has proved to be an excellent method of gas exchange in normal lungs in animals using lower MAP and rates of 1 to 20 Hz.[55-57] Whether this technique becomes a medical curiosity or represents a genuine advance in treatment of respiratory failure will depend upon determination of its effect on the diseased lung, initially in an animal model of lung injury.

After the initial experiments demonstrating the efficacy of gas exchange in animals with normal lungs the experiments of Thompson et al.[58] on dogs with oleic-acid-induced lung injury failed to demonstrate improved oxygenation with HFOV vs. conventional ventilation when MAP was matched with PEEP. In a similar study, Kolton et al.[59] compared conventional ventilation with HFO in oleic acid and lung lavage models of acute lung injury using matched MAP. In this study, they introduced a "sigh" maneuver (sustained inflation to 30 cm H_2O for 30 sec) in order to raise the lung above opening pressure before starting HFOV. Using this technique, they found an immediate and sustained improvement in PaO_2 as long as MAP was maintained above opening pressure. Animals maintained on CMV at MAP matched with HFOV died of hypoxaemia. In vitro plethysmography showed that the improved oxygenation coincided with substantially increased lung volumes in the group on HFOV. In a study by Hamilton et al.,[30] this sigh technique was applied to animals after lung lavage during both CMV and HFOV. Arterial oxygenation rose dramatically after a sigh in both groups;

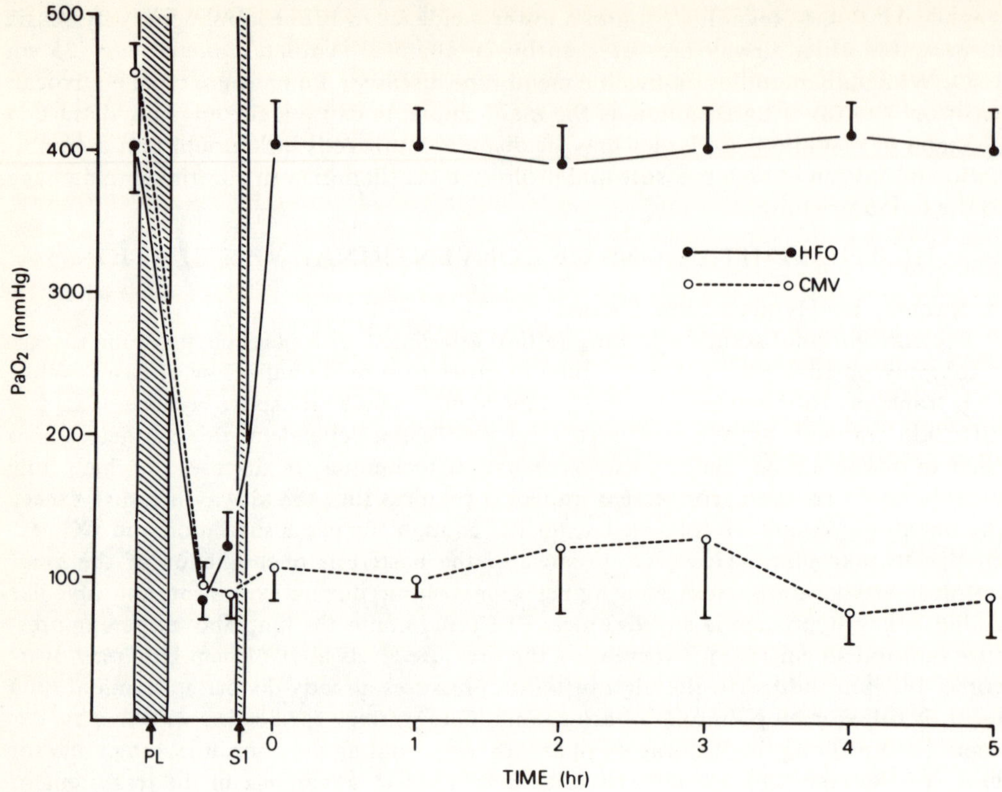

FIGURE 1. Comparison of HFO and CMV in a lung lavage model of lung injury. Both group are lavaged (PL) to produce a large A-a DO_2 on 100% oxygen. Initially there is no difference between the two groups until a sigh maneuver (S1) when PO_2 increases with HFOV but not with CMV. (From Hamilton et al., *J. Appl. Physiol.*, 55, 131, 1983. With permission.)

however, this improvement was not sustained in the CMV animals, which became hypoxic despite the application of PEEP. The HFOV animals maintained excellent oxygenation throughout the 5-hr study (Figure 1). Furthermore, microscopy showed a distinct difference in the lungs from the two other groups. CMV was associated with dense hyaline membrane formation while none was seen in these animals treated with HFOV (Figure 2).* Wright et al.[60] also using oleic-acid-induced lung injury in an animal model, demonstrated excellent gas exchange using HFOV; PaO_2 was determined by MAP dictated by the amount of fresh gas flow into the circuit, and CO_2 elimination was adjusted by altering the stroke volume delivered by the piston. Like Hamilton's group,[30] Wright et al. found that periodic hyperinflations or sigh maneuvers were required while animals were on HFOV in order to prevent atelectasis.

Several investigators are now examining the effect of HFOV on another manifestation of lung injury, with pulmonary edema. Using the lung lymph fistula model in sheep, Jefferies et al.[61] showed that lung lymph flow was unaffected by HFOV. More recently, Tamura et al.[62] have compared the effect of HFOV and CMV on lung water after pulmonary edema induced by starch emboli. Using the wet weight:dry weight ratio, they demonstrated significantly more edema associated with CMV. A striking difference was also seen in protein leak into the alveoli.

Using a similar method of HFOV in premature baboons, Truog et al.[63] compared gas exchange and pulmonary histology in experimental animals and a control group ventilated with CMV. They found improved oxygenation and CO_2 elimination with

* See Figure 2 after page 88.

lower MAP during HFOV over a 6-hr period, with no change in pulmonary phospholipid content of the lung between the two modes of ventilation.

Studies HFJV in animal models of lung injury are less numerous. Using an animal model of meconium aspiration, Mammel et al.[64] compared the effects of HFJV vs. CMV on oxygenation, pulmonary artery pressures (PAP), pulmonary vascular resistance, and intrapulmonary shunting (Qs:Qt). They found that pulmonary vascular resistance, PAP, and intrapulmonary shunting increased during HFJV and concluded that CMV was the superior mode of ventilation in this model. This finding may cast doubt on the use of HFJV, but HFOV clearly offers substantial advantages over CMV in terms of better gas exchange and less pulmonary damage in animal models of IRDS or acute lung injury. These animal studies suggest that HFOV is at least superior to CMV in the management of IRDS. In reality, HFOV is simply CPAP with the bonus of efficient CO_2 elimination. The concept in many ways resembles that used in the Kolobow et al.[65] technique of minimizing pulmonary bartorauma by using CPAP with an extracorporal membrane to eliminate CO_2.

V. HFV IN NEONATAL LUNG DISEASE

A. IRDS

Since human studies have established that HFOV can achieve excellent gas exchange in normal lungs[56,57] using lower MAP than CMV, this technique seemed logical for IRDS, where mechanical ventilation may contribute to ongoing pulmonary injury. In a preliminary study, Marchak et al.[66] used a variable-stroke piston pump to ventilate eight neonates with severe IRDS for 1 to 4 hr periods and compared the results with those from conventional mechanical ventilation. They found that with frequencies of 8 to 20 Hz and stroke volumes of 6 to 10 mℓ, they achieved better oxygenation and CO_2 elimination with HFOV. They were able to reduce the inspired oxygen substantially, and observed that arterial PO_2 varied with MAP, which in turn was adjusted by changes in fresh gas flow.

The same group[67] has extended this pilot study to 38 infants with severe hyaline membrane disease complicated by hypercarbia, ($PaCO_2 > 60$ mmHg), hypoxaemia (a:A ratio < 0.1), and high ventilatory pressures (MAP > 15 cm H_2O), and unresponsiveness to maximal ventilatory support. The infants were treated with HFOV using the same basic gas delivery system described by Marchak et al.[66] but with improved humidification and a safety "blow off" valve. This circuit allowed separate control of oxygenation in MAP and $PaCO_2$, by adjustments of stroke volume displacement of the piston. Oscillation was used for a period of 2 hr to 24 days (mean 3.3 days). In 14 of 18 infants treated successfully with HFOV (15 Hz), oxygenation improved immediately, with a rise in a:A ratio from 0.125 to 0.145 despite a reduction in the MAP from a mean of 19.3 cm H_2O on CMV to 16.2 H_2O on HFOV. The most striking improvement was in CO_2 elimination, with a reduction in mean $PaCO_2$ from 60 ± 18 mmHg to 37 ± 8 mmHg in of 3 hr. Successfully treated babies were then transferred back to CMV and weaned over 11 days (mean).

Frantz et al.[68] used HFO to treat 15 newborns with neonatal lung disease: 10 had IRDS and 5 had pulmonary interstitial emphysema. All had severe respiratory failure as evidenced by inspired oxygen requirements of greater than 40% and peak and inflation pressures of greater than 25 cm H_2O. This study used the Emerson high frequency ventilator, a rotary valve air-flow interruptor. In the 10 infants with IRDS, in whom oscillation was done for 1 hr, satisfactory gas exchange ($PaO_2 > 60$ mmHg; $PaCO_2 <$ 45 mm Hg) was maintained with lower peak inflation and MAP (measured inside the trachea) than those used with CMV. The five infants with severe pulmonary interstitial emphysema in whom improvement could not be achieved by reduced airway pressures on CMV and on rapid manual ventilation, were placed on HFOV as a last resort. With lower tracheal pressures on HFOV, two infants improved and were weaned from ventilatory support within 72 hr; a third required 26 days of HFOV before weaning. The remaining two died 48 hr after HFOV was begun. Of these five infants, four had marked increases in PO_2 and decreases in $PaCO_2$. Pokora et al.[69] have also used HFV in infants with pulmonary barotrauma. They ventilated a series of nine infants with either progressive pulmonary air leaks or bronchopleural fistulae secondary to IRDS or bacterial pneumonia using a HFJV. The air leaks diminished in seven of the nine infants, while arterial oxygenation improved in eight. In total, five survived. However, three of six infants who had HFJV for more than 20 hr developed tracheal obstruction. Of the nine infants, eight had an improvement in oxygenation. Boynton et al.[70] recently used a combination of HFOV and conventional ventilation in 12 infants dying of irreversible respiratory failure. Their series included a broad spectrum of neonatal lung disease, including congenital diaphragmatic hernia, IRDS with pulmonary interstitial emphysema, meconium aspiration, and pneumonia. In each case, $PaCO_2$ was significantly reduced and a:A ratio was increased when ventilation was changed to the HFO-CMV combination, while MAP were reduced. While four of the infants died (three with CDH and one with IRDS), six of the seven infants with pulmonary interstitial edema survived. Boynton et al.[70] have emphasized the importance of periodic lung inflations, as produced by CMV, in order to maintain lung volumes and prevent atelectasis in infants on HFOV.

These preliminary studies of the use of high frequency in neonates with IRDS and associated lung disease suggest that $PaCO_2$ can be controlled much more effectively by HFV than by CMV. Indeed, our experience indicates that hypocarbia is more of a concern than hypercarbia. The increase in PaO_2 is less impressive and less predictable but more favorable gas exchange can clearly be achieved with less pressure and thus less trauma to already damaged lungs.

VI. CONGENITAL DIAPHRAGMATIC HERNIA

Congenital diaphragmatic hernia represents an arrest in intrauterine lung development starting in the pseudoglandular period of fetal life (first 16 weeks). As all major airway branching occurs during this period, followed by alveolar development in the last trimester,[71] infants born with this condition have reduced airway branching and total alveolar number. This may be severe enough to be incompatible with life. Compounding this are the abnormalities of pulmonary vascular development that result in fetal circulation with right-to-left shunting. When this disease presents within the first 12 hr of life, mortality is about 50%. Most attention has been directed at pharmacological manipulations of pulmonary vascular tone; little emphasis has been placed on the effects of mechanical ventilation. Recently, we have identified a subgroup of infants with severe pulmonary hypoplasia characterized by severe hypoxemia and hypercarbia, who were unresponsive to vasodilator therapy;[72] we could not control $PaCO_2$ even with aggressive attempts at hyperventilation (ventilatory rates > 60/min, MAP > 23 cm H_2O). In 10 infants, changed to HFOV, $PaCO_2$ dropped immediately from a mean of 59 ± 5 mmHg to 27 ± 3 mmHg within 30 min, and this was achieved at substantially lower MAP (15 cm H_2O) (Figure 3).

Unfortunately, the increase in PaO_2 was less spectacular, with only a small unsustained improvement. Postmortem examination of the lungs revealed the reason. The first striking feature was dense hyaline membrane formation in infants who were mechanically ventilated. When the excised lungs were perfused with barium/gelatin suspension for detailed morphometric analysis, the total alveolar number was grossly less than that of normal newborns. The mean combined alveolar number for both lungs (from three infants) in this severely affected group[73] was 4 to 6×10^6, compared with 20×10^6 to 82×10^6 per lung in published normal controls series.[74,75] It is not surprising

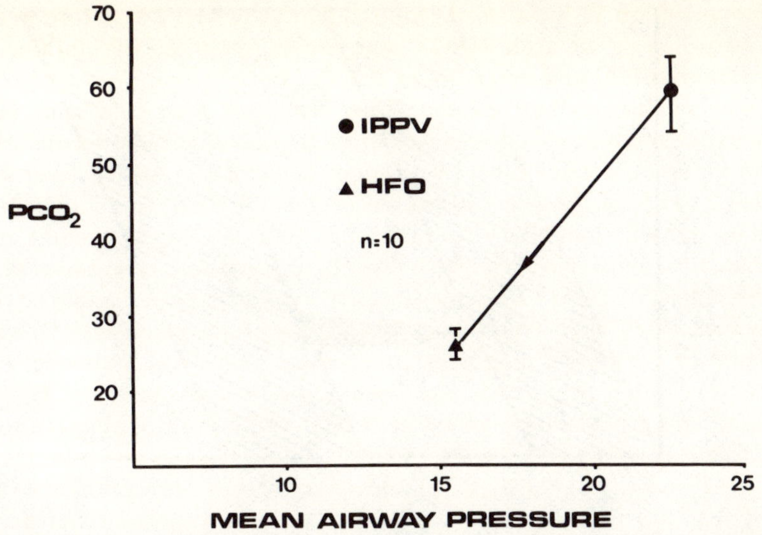

FIGURE 3. Change in $PaCO_2$ when changing from CMV (MAP > 20 cm H_2O, rate > 60/min) to HFOV in ten infants with congenital diphragmatic hernia. (From Bohn, D. J. et al., *J. Pediatr. Surg.*, 19, 666, 1984. With permission.)

then that these immature, hypoplastic lungs are susceptible to further damage with mechanical ventilation. We can now identify these patients early after repair of the diaphragmatic defect by examining the relationship between $PaCO_2$ and ventilatory parameters, and using this to determine whether or not to change to HFOV. Unfortunately, although we reversed the hypercarbia and acidosis in our ten infants, all died of progressive hypoxemia within 48 hr, suggesting that the degree of pulmonary hypoplasia was incompatible with life. Karl et al.[76] have used a similar technique of HFOV in five infants with congenital diaphragmatic hernia, using the Emerson model 2-VlV flow interrupter. Their experience was similar to ours; CO_2 control was rapidly re-established by HFOV, but little change occurred in oxygenation. In a more recent study of three infants with congenital diaphragmatic hernia, HFOV superimposed on conventional intermittent mandatory ventilation resulted in only one survivor.

HFOV has also proved effective in the management of infants with persistent fetal circulation in which hyperventilation and respiratory alkalosis can reverse the right-to-left shunting. Hypocarbia can be readily induced by HFOV; indeed, frequently, the problem is an excessively low $PaCO_2$, even at low airway pressures.

VII. HEMODYNAMIC EFFECTS ON HFV

The hemodynamic effects of HFV have been documented in human and animal studies[55,61,77] showing no change in cardiac output when CMV is switched to HFOV. Jefferies et al.[61] have measured mean PAP in animals, and documented no change between CMV and HFOV. Gioia et al.[77] also noted no changes in pulmonary arterial pressure during HFV, whereas Bland et al.[32] in a study using lambs showed a small increase from 22 ± 2 mmHg to 27 ± 4 mmHg in mean PAP.

The only published study on hemodynamic effects on HFV in children is that of Vincent et al.,[79] who used HFOV (Emerson flow interrupter) in a group of six infants (1 to 8-months-old) who were being electively ventilated after cardiac surgery for correction of congenital heart defects. After the switch from CMV to HFOV, the PAP rose from 20 ± 2 mmHg to 22 ± 2 mmHg, associated with a rise in pulmonary vascular

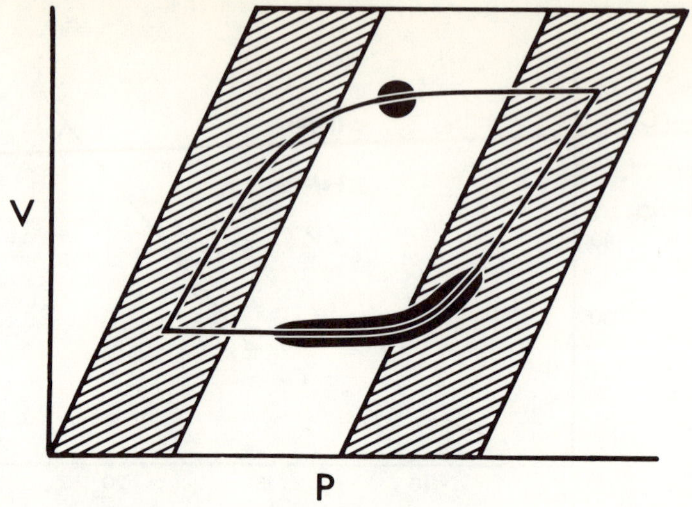

FIGURE 4. Strategy for HFOV in hypoxic lung disease. The P.V. curve of the lung is bounded by a band of opening pressure and a band of closing pressure. The circle represents the optimum position for HFV.

resistance. At the same time, $PaCO_2$ rose from 39 to 43 mmHg, which would explain the increase in PAP. Cardiac output did not change with the different modes of ventilation. HFOV was used with these infants for only 1-hr periods.

More extended investigation of the hemodynamic effects of HFV is needed, particularly in the pulmonary vascular system. In theory, it could be of considerable benefit in children who have congenital heart disease associated with a reactive pulmonary vascular bed, (e.g., ventricular septal defect, transposition of the great vessels, total anomolus pulmonary venous drainage, and children who have had Fontans procedure where changes in pulmonary vascular resistance can directly affect morbidity). A method of ventilation that avoids large cyclical pressure swings, which affect the intra-aveolar pulmonary capillaries, may have a significant impact on pulmonary vascular resistance.

VIII. HFOV IN NEONATAL RESPIRATORY FAILURE

A. Strategy for Hypoxic Lung Disease

Bryan has recently proposed a strategy of "opening" the atelectatic lung by a sustained sigh maneuver, to increase oxygenation and reduce airway pressures.[80] This concept is based on the animal experiments of Hamilton et al.,[30] who showed that oxygenation could be improved in their model of hyaline membrane disease only by opening the lung by "sighing" the animals. This requires a completely different HFOV strategy.

In the atelectatic lung, increased airway pressure is required to open closed lung units. With each ventilator stroke, no volume change occurs in the lung until opening pressure is exceeded, after which there will be rapid alveolar recruitment (Figure 4). During expiration there will be derecruitment back to the original atelectatic state as closing pressure is reached, after which no further gas exchange occurs. Therefore, gas is exchanged only in late inspiration and early expiration. Furthermore, the cyclic distention and collapse of terminal lung units causes additional parenchymal damage. The strategy with HFOV is to raise the lung above opening pressure with a sustained infla-

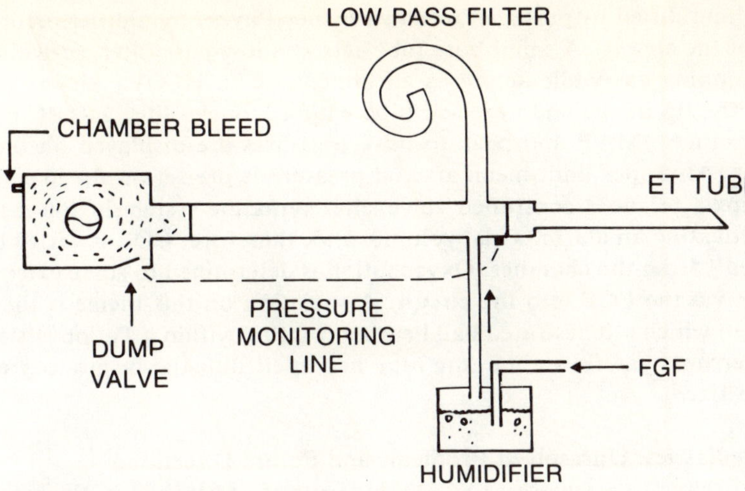

FIGURE 5. Diagramatic representation of the high frequency oscillation system currently in use. Stroke volume (CO_2 control) can be altered by adjusting the chamber "bleed" while MAP (oxygenation) is adjusted by FGF.

tion maneuver to 30 cm H_2O, thereby regaining lost lung volume. This favorable position on the PV curve is maintained with HFOV, which, since airway pressure is not allowed to fall, holds lung volume constant. This open-lung strategy interrupts the vicious cycle of atelectasis and falling lung compliance that lead to increased positive pressure and further lung damage.

B. HFV: Gas Delivery Systems

Some confusion exists over what constitutes HFV, or when ventilation ceases to be conventional and can be classified as HFV. Froese[81] has proposed that the term be reserved for techniques that exceed four times the normal frequency; rather than referring to HFOV and HFJV, one should use the generic terms HFV-A for systems that depend on active expiration and HFV-P for those in which expiration is passive. This would help reduce the confusing terminology that is currently applied to different systems. Both systems are used in pediatric intensive care, but the principles involved differ greatly.

C. HFV: Passive Expiration (HFJV)

Although many varieties of jet ventilators are currently in use, the principle of operation is basically the same. The ventilator is driven by a high pressure gas source (50 psi) with a pressure regulator incorporated into the system in order to adjust the driving pressure over the range 5 to 50 psi. Small volumes of high frequency insufflations are delivered via a small-bore catheter within the airway. The inspiratory time can be varied with either fluidics or a magnetically controlled solenoid valve. Inspired gases are mixed by a blender but air entrainment is common.

D. HFV: Active Expiration (HFOV)

Considerable experience with the use of HFOV in neonatal respiratory failure has now been accumulated and it has proved to be a safe and reliable form of HFV. The circuit used in our institution resembles the one originally described in many respects, but with some added safety features (Figure 5). The piston pump is driven by a high-speed electric motor. Stroke-volume displacement is varied by allowing a "bleed" of compressed gas from the chamber. Fresh gas flow (FGF) of oxygen/air mixture (5 to

15 ℓ/min) is humidified by passage through a Fisher-Paykel humidifier before delivery to the peak of the airway. A small-bore tube acts as a low-pass filter, providing an exit for CO_2-containing gas while acting as an impedance to HFOV. Airway pressure is measured at the tip of the endotracheal tube with a Honeywell® 140 PC differential pressure transducer; MAP and peak-to-peak pressures are displayed on the body of the ventilator. An upper limit mean arterial pressure is pre-set on the machine: if exceeded, it trips a solenoid-controlled valve, that vents the system in 100 msec, at the same time activating an alarm. Tidal volume, and, therefore, CO_2, is varied by adjusting the "bleed" from the chamber. Oxygenation is determined to some extent by varying the MAP via the FGF into the circuit. A variation on this theme is the Emerson rotating ball in which a fenestrated ball bearing rotating within a Teflon® sleeve intermittently interrupts gas flow. The rate may be varied, but the inspiratory:expiratory ratio remains fixed.

E. HFV in Pediatrics: Unresolved Problems and Future Directions

While HFV may prove superior to CMV in terms of gas exchange, the high frequencies and gas flows used will probably preclude any superiority in terms of technical safety. This reflects more on the industry's inability to keep pace with medical advances than on HFV itself. Both HFJV and HFOV require rapid-response venting systems in case of a malfunction which would cause lung rupture. The HFOV circuit, which uses no moving valves, appears intrinsically safer in this respect. With HFJV using rapid rates (> 15 Hz), the decrease in expiratory time leads to an inadvertent PEEP with a fall in cardiac output.[82] An increase in lung volume has also been reported recently with the use of HFOV in human patients.[83] Indeed both systems suffer somewhat from the inability to determine precisely what alveolar pressure is. Perhaps the only way to measure true alveolar pressure is by the airway occlusion technique. Attempts to measure intratracheal pressure are fraught with difficulty due to artificial readings caused by the Bernoulli effect on the catheter. In neither system can humidification be described as completely satisfactory due to the high gas flows. With HFOV the inspired gas can be humidified with a heated water humidifier, while HFJV relies on entrainment of moisture from a reservoir or infusion of droplets into the inspired line. Little information is available on muco-ciliary transport in the lung with HFV, although one study by McEvoy et al.[84] suggests that muco-ciliary transport is diminshed during HFOV. During extensive clinical use in neonatal ventilation, blockage of endotracheal tubes has not been a problem.

Advances in the treatment of respiratory failure in neonates in the past 20 years have contributed considerably to the reduction we have seen in neonatal mortality. Perhaps the greatest strides have been taken in the treatment of IRDS, first with the introduction of mechanical ventilation in the 1960s and then with CPAP in the 1970s. Will the 1980s be the decade when HFV becomes the accepted mode of treatment for this disease, or will the development of artificial surfactant make mechanical ventilation of any type obsolete?

Little doubt remains that mechanical ventilation worsens lung damage in any form of acute lung injury, whether in children or adults. In infants, the mortality remains unacceptably high; 40% of infants with IRDS < 1000 die of respiratory failure while about 30% of surviving infants develop chronic lung disease. So, although mechanical ventilation represents a great advance in the treatment of this disease, it remains part of the problem.

Even though dramatic improvements in IRDS have been reported with artificial surfactant, these are unpredictable and frequently not sustained. Short term improvements in oxygenation do not resolve the problem of primary surfactant deficiency or the need for positive pressure ventilation, which will further damage the lung. A combination of artificial surfactant and HFV may well be the answer.

REFERENCES

1. Northway, W. H., Jr., Rosan, R. C., and Porter, D. Y., Pulmonary disease following respirator therapy of hyaline membrane disease: bronchopulmonary dysplasia, *N. Engl. J. Med.*, 276, 357, 1967.
2. Edwards, D. K., Dyer, W. M., and Northway, W. H., Twelve years experience with bronchopulmonary dysplasia, *Pediatrics,* 59, 839, 1977.
3. Bancalari, E., Abdenour, E. E., Feller, R., and Bannon, J., Bronchopulmonary dysplasia: clinical presentation, *J. Pediatr.*, 95, 819, 1979.
4. Tooley, W. H., Epidemiology of bronchopulmonary dysplasia, *J. Pediatr.*, 95, 815, 1979.
5. Bland, R. D., Kim, M. H., and Woodson, J. L., High frequency mechanical ventilation in severe hyaline membrane disease: an alternative treatment, *Crit. Care Med.*, 8, 275, 1980.
6. Roussos, C. and Macklem, P., The respiratory muscles, *N. Engl. J. Med.*, 786, 307, 1982.
7. Benson, F. and Celander, O., Respirator treatment of severe pulmonary insufficiency in the newborn infant, *Acta Paediatr. Scan.*, Suppl. 48, 118, 1959.
8. Gregory, G. A., Kitterman, J. A., Phibbs, R. H., Hamilton, W. K., and Tooley, W. H., Treatment of idiopathic respiratory distress syndrome with continuous positive airway pressure, *N. Engl. J. Med.*, 284, 1330, 1971.
9. Lauweryns, J. M., Hyaline membrane disease: a pathological study of 55 infants, *Arch. Dis. Child.*, 40, 618, 1965.
10. Lauweryns, J. M., Hyaline membrane disease in newborn infants. Macroscopic, radiographic and light and electron microscopic studies, *Hum. Pathol.*, 1, 175, 1970.
11. Gandy, G., Jacobson, W., and Gairdner, D., Hayline membrane disease I: cellular changes, *Arch. Dis. Child.*, 45, 289, 1970.
12. Finlay-Jones, J., Papdimitriou, J. M., and Barter, R. A., Pulmonary hayline membrane: light and electron microscopic study of the early stage, *J. Pathol.*, 112, 117, 1974.
13. Coalson, J. J., Pathophysiologic features of respiratory distress in the infant and adult, in Critical Care, State of the Art, Critical Care Medicine, Denver, Colo., 1982.
14. Desa, D. J., Pulmonary fluid content in infants with respiratory distress, *J. Pathol.*, 97, 469, 1969.
15. Rudolph, A. M., Drorbaugh, J. E., Auld, P. A. M., et al., Studies on the circulation in the neonatal period: the circulation in respiratory distress syndrome, *Pediatrics,* 27, 551, 1961.
16. Nilsson, R., The artificially ventilated preterm rabbit neonate as experimental model of hyaline membrane disease, *Acta Anaesth. Scand.*, 26, 89, 1982.
17. McAdams, A. J., Coen, R., Kleinman, L. I., Tsang, R., and Sutherland, J., The experimental production of hyaline membranes in premature rhesus monkeys, *Am. J. Pathol.*, 70, 277, 1973.
18. Ogden, B. E., Murphy, S. A., Saunders, G. C., and Johnson, J. D., Lung lavage of newborns with respiratory distress syndrome (RDS): prolonged neutrophil influx is associated with bronchopulmonary dysplasia (BPD), *Am. Rev. Resp. Dis.*, 121, 194, 1980.
19. Merritt, T. A., Puccia, J., and Stuard, I. D., Cytologic evaluation of pulmonary effluent in neonates with respiratory distress syndrome and bronchopulmonary dysplasia, *Acta Cytol.*, 25, 631, 1982.
20. Barter, R. A., Finlay-Jones, L., and Walters, M., Pulmonary hyaline membranes: sites of formation in adult lungs after assisted respiration and inhalation of oxygen, *J. Pathol. Bacteriol.*, 95, 481, 1968.
21. Capers, T. H., Pulmonary hyaline membrane formation in the adult, *Am. J. Med.*, 31, 701, 1963.
22. Pratt, P. C., Vollmer, R. T., Shelbourne, J. D., and Crapo, J. D., Pulmonary morphology in a multihospital collaborative extracorporeal membrane oxygenation project. I. light microscopy, *Am. J. Pathol.*, 95, 191, 1979.
23. Avery, M. E. and Mead, J., Surface properties in relation to atelectasis and hyaline membrane disease, *Am. J. Dis. Child.*, 97, 517, 1959.
24. Gairdner, D., Marks, J., Roscoe, J. D., and Brettell, R. O., The fluid shift from the vascular compartment immediately after birth, *Arch. Dis. Child.*, 33, 489, 1958.
25. Tannenberg, J., Fetal and postnatal atelectasis: factors essential in initiating spontaneous respiration and the significance of hyaline membrane formation in the newborn, *Am. J. Clin. Pathol.*, 32, 306, 1959.
26. Lieberman, J. and Kellogg, F., A deficiency of pulmonary fibrinolysis in hyaline or membrane disease, *N. Engl. J. Med.*, 262, 999, 1960.
27. Liebeberman, J., Clinical syndromes associated with deficient fibrinolytic activity. I. New concept of hyaline membrane disease, *N. Engl. J. Med.*, 260, 619, 1959.
28. Nash, G., Blennerhassett, J. B., and Pontoppidan, H., Pulmonary lesions associated with oxygen therapy and artificial ventilation, *N. Eng. J. Med.*, 262, 368, 1967.
29. Schwieler, G. H. and Robertson, B., Liquid ventilation in newborn rabbits, *Biol. Neonate,* 29, 343, 1976.

30. Hamilton, P. P., Adebusola, O., Smith, J., Gillan, J. E., Cutz, E., Froese, A. B., and Bryan, A. C., Comparison of conventional and high frequency ventilation: oxygenation and lung pathology, *J. Appl. Physiol.*, 55, 131, 1983.
31. Bressack, M. A. and Bland, R. D., Alveolar hypoxia increases lung fluid filtration in unanesthetised newborn lambs, *Circ. Res.*, 46, 111, 1980.
32. Bland, R. D., Bressack, M. A., Haberkern, C. M., and Hansen, T. N., Lung fluid balance in hypoxic awake newborn lambs and mature sheep, *Biol. Neonate*, 38, 221, 1980.
33. Hansen, T. N., Haberkern, C. M., Hazinski, T. A., and Bland, R. D., Lung field balance in hypoxic lambs, *Pediatr. Res.*, 18, 434, 1984.
34. Egan, E. A., Dillon, W. P., and Zorn, S., Fetal lung liquid absorption and alveolar epithelial solute permeability in surfactant deficient, breathing fetal lambs, *Pediatr. Res.*, 18, 566, 1984.
35. Jobe, A., Ikegami, M., Jacobs, H., Jones, S., and Conaway, D., Permeability of premature lamb lungs to protein and the effect of surfactant on that permeability, *J. Appl. Physiol.*, 55, 169, 1983.
36. Jefferies, A. L., Coates, G., and O'Brodovich, H., Pulmonary epithelial permeability in hyaline disease, *N. Engl. J. Med.*, 311, 1075, 1984.
37. Kudoh, I., Effect of mechanical ventilation on lung water volume in dogs, *Crit. Care Med.*, 12, 443, 1984.
38. Lambertson, C. J., Effects of oxygen at high partial pressures, in *Handbook of Physiology*, Vol. 2, Section 3, Fenn, W. O. and Rahn, H., Eds., Williams & Wilkins, Baltimore, 1965.
39. De Lemos, R., Wolfsdorf, J., Nachman, R., Block, A., Leiby, G., Wilkinson, H. A., Allen, T., Haller, J. A., Morgan, W., and Avery, M. E., Lung injury from oxygen in lambs: the role of artificial ventilation, *Anesthesiology*, 30, 608, 1969.
40. Ahlstrom, H., Pulmonary mechanics in infants surviving severe respiratory insufficiency, *Acta Paediatr. Scand.*, 64, 69, 1975.
41. Lamarre, A., Linsao, L., Reilly, B. J., Swyer, P. R., and Levison, H., Residual pulmonary abnormalities in survivors of idiopathic respiratory distress syndrome, *Am. Rev. Resp. Dis.*, 108, 56, 1973.
42. Clark, J. M. and Lambertson, C. J., Pulmonary oxygen toxicity: review, *Pharmacol. Rev.*, 23, 37, 1971.
43. Ludwin, S. K., Northway, W. H., Jr., and Benschk, G., Oxygen toxicity in the newborn: necrotising bronchiolitis in mice exposed to 100% oxygen, *Lab. Invest.*, 5, 425, 1974.
44. Bonikos, D. S., Bensch, K. G., and Northway, W. H., Oxygen toxicity in the newborn, *Am. J. Pathol.*, 85, 623, 1976.
45. Escobedo, M. B., Robotham, J. L., Hilliard, J. L., Smith, F. R., Meredith, K., Johnson, D., Coalson, J. J., Walsh, W., and Kuehl, T. J., The preterm baboon with hyaline membrane disease as a model for bronchopulmonary dysplasia, *Pediatr. Res.*, 15, 718, 1981.
46. Rhodes, P. G., Hall, R. T., and Leonidas, J. C., Chronic pulmonary disease in neonates with assisted ventilation, *Paediatrics*, 55, 788, 1975.
47. Edwards, D. K., Dyer, W. H., and Northway, W. H., Jr., Twelve years experience with bronchopulmonary dysplasia, *Pediatrics*, 59, 839, 1979.
48. Taghizadeh, A. and Reynolds, E. O. R., Pathogenesis of bronchopulmonary dysplasia following hyaline membrane disease, *Am. J. Pathol.*, 82, 241, 1976.
49. Reynolds, E. O. R. and Taghizadeh, A., Improved prognosis of infants mechanically ventilated for hyaline membrane disease, *Arch. Dis. Child.*, 49, 505, 1974.
50. Phillip, A. G. S., Oxygen plus pressure plus time: the etiology of bronchopulmonary dysplasia, *Pediatrics*, 55, 44, 1975.
51. Stocks, J. and Godfrey, S., The role of artificial ventilation, oxygen and CPAP in the pathogenesis of lung damage in neonates: assessment by serial measurements of lung function, *Pediatrics*, 57, 352, 1976.
52. Bryan, A. C., *High Frequency Ventilation in the Therapy of Respiratory Distress Syndrome*, Raivio, K. O., Hallman, N., Kouvalainen, K., and Valimak, I., Eds., Academic, New York, 1984, 249.
53. Reynolds, E. O. R., Effect of alterations in mechanical ventilator settings for mechanical ventilation in severe hyaline membrane disease, *Arch. Dis. Child.*, 46, 152, 1971.
54. Boros, S. J., Variations in inspiratory-expiratory ration and airway pressure waveform during mechanical ventilation: the significance of mean airway pressure, *J. Pediatr.*, 94, 114, 1979.
55. Bohn, D. J., Miyasaka, K., Marchak, B. E., Thompson, W. K., Froese, A. B., and Bryan, A. C., Ventilation by high frequency oscillation, *J. Appl. Physiol.*, 48, 710, 1980.
56. Butler, W. J., Bohn, D. J., Bryan, A. C., and Froese, A. B., Ventilation by frequency oscillation in humans, *Anesth. Analg.*, 59, 577, 1980.
57. Goldstein, D., Slutsky, A. S., Ingram, R., Westerman, P., Venegas, J., and Drazen, J., CO_2 elimination by high frequency ventilation (4—10 Hz) in normal subjects, *Am. Rev. Respir. Dis.*, 123, 251, 1981.
58. Thompson, W. K., Marchak, B. E., Froese, A. B., and Bryan, A. C., High frequency oscillation compared with standard ventilation in pulmonary injury model, *J. Appl. Physiol.*, 55, 543, 1982.

59. Kolton, M., Cattran, C. B., Kent, G., Voleyesi, G., Froese, A. B., and Bryan, A. C., Oxygenation during high frequency ventilation compared with conventional mechanical ventilation in two models of lung injury, *Anesth. Analg.*, 61, 323, 1982.
60. Wright, K., Lyrene, R. K., Truog, W. E., Standaert, T. A., Murphy, J., and Woodrum, D. E., Ventilation by high frequency oscillation in rabbits with oleic acid lung disease, *J. Appl. Physiol.*, 50, 1056, 1981.
61. Jefferies, A. L., Hamilton, P., and Bryan, A. C., Effect of high frequency oscillation on lung lymph flow, *J. Appl. Physiol.*, 55, 1373, 1983.
62. Tamura, M., Kawano, T., and Bryan, A. C., The effect of high frequency oscillation and conventional mechanical ventilation on extravascular lung water, *Clin. Invest. Med.*, 7, 85, 1984.
63. Truog, W. E., Standaert, T. A., Murphy, J., Palmer, S., Woodrum, D. E., and Hodson, W. A., Effect of high-frequency oscillation on gas exchange and pulmonary phospholipids in experimental hyaline membrane disease, *Am. Rev. Respir. Dis.*, 127, 585, 1983.
64. Mammel, M. C., Gordon, M. J., Connett, J. E., and Boros, S. J., Comparison of high-frequency jet ventilation and conventional mechanical ventilation in meconium aspiration model, *J. Pediatr.*, 103, 630, 1983.
65. Kolobow, T., Gattinoni, L., and Tomlinson, T., An alternative to breathing, *J. Thorac. Cardiovas. Surg.*, 75, 261, 1978.
66. Marchak, B. E., Thompson, W. K., Duffty, P., Miyaki, T., Bryan, M. H., Bryan, A. C., and Froese, A. B., Treatment of RDS by high frequency oscillatory ventilation: a preliminary report, *J. Pediatr.*, 99, 287, 1981.
67. Tamura, M., Toshio, K., Fitzjames, I., and Bryan, A. C., High frequency oscillation in neonates with terminal respiratory insufficiency, in preparation.
68. Frantz, I. D., Werthammer, J., and Stark, A. R., High frequency ventilation in premature infants with lung disease: adequate gas exchange at low tracheal pressure, *Pediatrics*, 71, 483, 1983.
69. Pokora, T., Bing, D., Mammel, M., and Boros, S., Neonatal high frequency ventilation, *Pediatrics*, 72, 27, 1983.
70. Boynton, B. R., Mannino, F. L., Davis, R. F., Kopotic, R. J., and Guillermo, F., Combined high-frequency oscillatory ventilation and intermittent mandatory ventilation in critically ill neonates, *J. Pediatr.*, 105, 297, 1984.
71. Ried, L., The lung: its growth and remodeling in health and disease, *Am. J. Roentgenol.*, 129, 777, 1977.
72. Bohn, D. J., James, I., Filler, R. M., Ein, S. H., Wesson, D. E., Shandling, B., Stephens, C., and Barker, G. A., The relationship between $PaCO_2$ and ventilation parameters in predicting survival in congenital diaphragmatic hernia, *J. Pediatr. Surg.*, 19, 666, 1984.
73. Bohn, D. J., Rabinovitch, M., Tamura, M., Bryan, A. C., and Barker, G. A., The relationship between $PaCO_2$ and ventilatory parameters in predicting mortality in congenital diaphragmatic hernia, *Am. Rev. Respir. Dis.*, 129, A212, 1984.
74. Dunnhill, M. S., Postnatal growth of the lung, *Thorax*, 17, 329, 1962.
75. Hislop, A. and Fairweather, D. V. I., Alveolar number and size in the human fetal and neonatal lung, *Am. Rev. Resp. Dis.*, 129, A208, 1984.
76. Karl, S. R., Ballantine, T. V. N., and Snider, M. T., High frequency ventilation at rates of 375 to 1800 cycles per minute in four neonates with congenital diaphragmatic hernia, *J. Pediatr. Surg.*, 18, 822, 1983.
77. Gioia, F. R., Rinehart, G., and Traystam, R. J., Regional and lobar pulmonary blood flow with high frequency ventilation, *Pediatr. Res.*, 15, 719, 1981.
78. Bland, R. D., Usha, Raj. J., Hazinski, T. A., Sedin, G. E., and Goldberg, R. B., Lung fluid balance in lambs, *Pediatr. Res.*, 16, 280A, 1982.
79. Vincent, R. N., Stark, A. R., Land, P., Close, R. H., Norwood, W. I., Castaneda, A. R., and Frantz, I. D., Haemodynamic response to high frequency ventilation in infants following cardiac surgery, *Pediatrics*, 73, 426, 1984.
80. Bryan, A. C., High frequency ventilation and oscillatory techniques in the treatment of respiratory distress syndrome, in *Pulmonary Surfactant System*, Cosmi, E. V. and Scarpelli, E. M., Eds., Elsevier, Amsterdam, 1983, 143.
81. Froese, A. B., High frequency ventilation — a critical assessment, in *Critical Care — State of the Art*, Shoemaker, W. E., Ed., W. B. Saunders, Philadelphia, 1984, 5.
82. Fusciardi, J., Rouby, J. J., Benhamou, D., and Viars, P., Haemodynamic consequences of increasing mean airway pressure during high frequency jet ventilation, *Chest*, 66, 31, 1984.
83. Saari, A. F., Rossing, T. H., Solway, J., and Drazen, J. M., Lung inflation during high frequency ventilation, *Am. Rev. Respir. Dis.*, 129, 333, 1984.
84. McEvoy, R. D. and Davies, N. J. H., Hedenstierna. Lung muco-ciliary transport during high frequency ventilation, *Am. Rev. Respir. Dis.*, 126, 452, 1982.
85. Cutz, E., Personal communication.

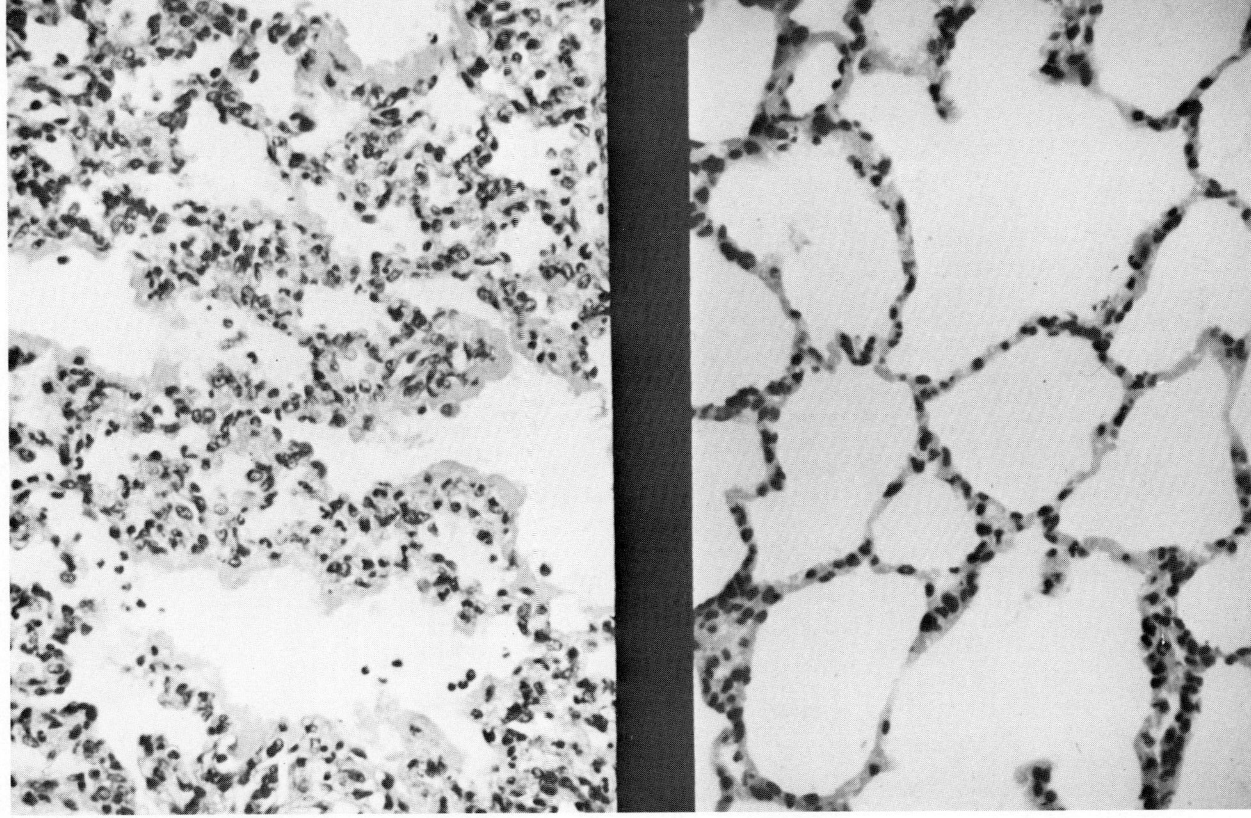

FIGURE 2. Comparison of postmortem microscopic specimens in lung lavage model after 5 hr of HFOV (right panel) and CMV (left panel). Note the severe hyaline membrane formation with CMV. (From Hamilton et al., *J. Appl. Physiol.*, 55, 131, 1983. With permission.)

Chapter 8

DELIVERY EQUIPMENT AND MONITORING TECHNIQUES FOR HIGH FREQUENCY VENTILATION

Charles K. Waterson and Stuart F. Quan

TABLE OF CONTENTS

I. INTRODUCTION

Mechanical ventilation at high rates (<60 c/min) places special constraints on equipment design and operation. Ventilation at these higher rates is accompanied by increased flow and pressure transients. The compliance of the breathing circuit and the compression of gases in the ventilator and airway become increasingly important. The design of delivery systems for HFV must take these special considerations into account while maintaining the simplicity and reliability necessary for clinical life-support equipment. Monitoring the effectiveness of gas exchange with HFV is also different — and perhaps more difficult — than with conventional rates and volumes. This chapter will discuss present HFV system designs and address some of these special concerns. When relevant, the physics of gas flow and lung mechanics will be considered as each affects the design or operation of a high frequency ventilator. Also included is a brief synopsis of the regulatory status of HFV ventilators in the U.S.

II. HFV DELIVERY SYSTEMS

A. Classification of HFV Delivery Systems

Many different methodologies have been devised for deliverying HFV. The number of design variations approximates the number of investigators in the field. The only features held in common are operation at ventilatory frequencies above the normal physiologic range for spontaneous breathing and reduced peak inspiratory airway pressures. Furthermore, not all investigators have fully characterized their HFV delivery systems. In addition, there is no general agreement about what measurements are necessary to adequately describe HFV methodology. There is a need to categorize HFV systems on the basis of design or physiologic effect. By examining the general approach to HFV taken in a specific ventilator design, and considering the gas flow mechanics it attempts to exploit, it is possible to assign systems to groups with similar features. The problem with this approach is that each technique within a group may exploit slightly different mechnical factors and have different characteristics governing its effectiveness. Because of this, delivery systems with apparently similar design may be grouped together, but care must be used in extrapolating results obtained with a particular system to all in the same group.

Several schemes have been proposed for categorizing the many different techniques used to deliver HFV. Some classifications are based solely on ventilatory frequency. Other categorizations depend on how the gas flow is delivered to the airway. Froese considered whether expiration was an active or a passive process to define two broad categories, called high-frequency ventilation — active expiration (HVF-A) and high-frequency ventilation — passive expiration (HFV-P).[1] In this chapter, a functional classification system is used. Under that system, the three major divisions are HFPPV, HFJV, and HFOV. Externally applied chest compressions and infrasonic vibrations also have been used experimentally, and will constitute a fourth division, HFBSO. Several characteristics of the ventilator and breathing circuit are used to categorize a ventilator into one of the major groups. These characteristics include the effective frequency range, whether expiration is an active or passive process, whether inspiration is an active or passive process, whether or not entrainment of gases is allowed, whether the system is volume or pressure limited, whether or not an expiratory valve is used, how the gas flow is derived and controlled, and where the ventilatory gas flow is introduced to the airway or breathing circuit. To avoid any confusion, definitions for some of the terms used to describe these ventilator characteristics will be provided here.

Expiration is considered to be passive when it occurs as a result of the elastic recoil of the chest wall and lung. This is the case in conventional positive-pressure ventilation and SB. However, when the expiratory phase of a ventilator causes a negative (subatmospheric) airway pressure, expiration is considered to be an active process. By the same reasoning, active inspiration is caused by either a positive pressure applied to the airway or a negative pressure applied to the exterior of the chest. Passive inspiration occurs when the chest has been actively collapsed and re-expands due to elastic recoil. Such may be the case with externally applied chest compressions.

Entrainment of gas occurs when a jet or column of gas moving at a high velocity drags the surrounding gas along with it. This phenomena is governed by the conservation of momentum and energy. When a given mass of fluid exits a nozzle at high speed it contains an amount of momentum and energy which is directly proportional to the mass of fluid and the velocity at which it is traveling. Friction between the fluid in the jet and the stationary fluid around it causes some of the stationary fluid to be accelerated and some of the high speed fluid to decelerate. In order for the total amount of momentum and energy in the moving fluid to be constant (it must remain constant since momentum and energy cannot be destroyed or created), more fluid must now be moving, but at a lower velocity. More mass has been recruited into the fluid stream, but at the expense of overall velocity. This will continue until all available gas is moving at a uniform, lower speed or until some other momentum or energy source, such as a pressure gradient, causes a change in gas velocity.[2] Obviously, if there is no source of entrainment gas, the jet will continue at a high velocity. Likewise, if a great deal of entrainment occurs, the jet will slow down quickly. It should also be clear that the amount of entrainment can be affected by a multitude of factors, such as the size of the jet, the velocity of the jet, and the ease by which surrounding gases can be recruited and accelerated.[3-10]

Most high frequency ventilators are time-cycled. However, they vary with respect to whether a constant volume is delivered to the airway during the inspiratory phase. In many designs, termed open systems, there is no exhalation valve to prevent the escape of gas through the expiratory pathway during inspiration. These designs depend either on delivering gas to the airway more rapidly than it can exhaust or exploiting properties of fluid mechanics to control inspiratory flow. Entrainment and spontaneous ventilation are possible with open systems. Other designs, termed closed systems, employ valves to limit exhaust during inspiration and to prevent entrainment. Spontaneous ventilation is not usually possible. Because of the pressure gradients caused by the rapid gas flows and high ventilatory rates, pressure controlled HFV is not common.

Gas flow in HFV systems can be derived in two ways. The most common approach is to use a high-pressure source, such as the hospital piped gas supply, directly. The gas is blended to the desired concentration and may be heated and humidified. It is regulated to a prescribed pressure inside the ventilator and a valve periodically opens, to allow it to be delivered to the breathing circuit. The other approach uses a piston, diaphragm, or loudspeaker to produce pressure and volume changes in the airway while the fresh gas is washed through the system as a steady bias flow.

Several different locations in the breathing circuit and airway are used for the introduction of ventilatory gas flows in HFV. For ease of classification, the trachea near the carina will be considered the distal airway; the top (connector end) of the endotracheal tube will be the proximal airway; and the rest of the endotracheal tube, or the trachea just below the vocal cords if no endotracheal tube is used, will be the middle airway.

B. HFPPV

HFPPV originated from attempts to abolish interference from respiratory artifacts in physiological studies of carotid sinus nerve activity.[11-13] It was theorized that these artifacts could be reduced by employing increasingly smaller tidal volumes at higher

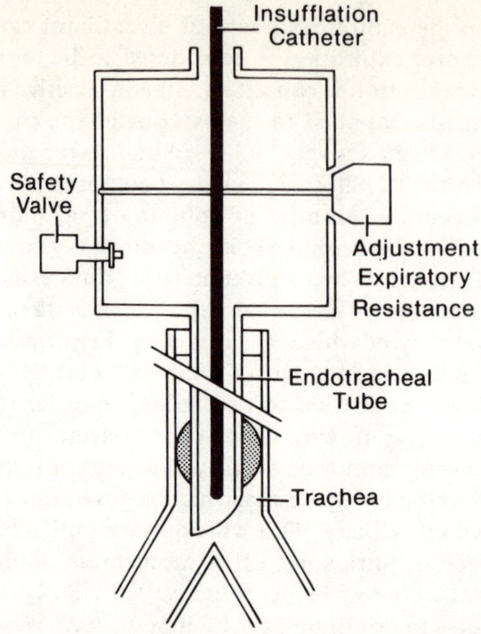

FIGURE 1. Schematic diagram of the insufflation catheter for HFPPV. There is no low-resistance source for entrainment and no expiratory valve to prevent escape of gas during insufflation. (From Heijman, K., Heijman, I., Jonzon, A., et al., *Acta Anaesth. Scand.*, 16, 176, 1972. With permission.)

than normal ventilatory rates. The goal was to maintain a constant effective minute ventilation while reducing the fluctuations in airway and intrapleural pressures associated with positive-pressure ventilation. When rates of 60 c/min (1 Hz) were used with special ventilators having small internal compressible volumes, it was found that adequate gas exchange could be maintained with tidal volumes which approached anatomic dead space volumes. Currently, HFPPV generally refers to time-cycled flow-generating techniques used at ventilatory frequencies above those associated with normal spontaneous breathing. Either conventional ventilators or special devices to deliver gas to the proximal airway without allowing entrainment or exploiting jet flow properties may be employed for HFPPV.[12-20] Inspiration is active and expiration is a passive process. A wide range of ventilatory rates, as high as 1320 c/min (22 Hz), have been reported.[21] However, frequencies between 60 c/min (1 Hz) and 120 c/min (2 Hz) are most common.

1. Methods of Generating and Controlling HFPPV

A ventilator to be used for HFPPV must either be capable of producing sufficiently high inspiratory flow rates to fill internal compressible volumes and deliver adequate tidal volume within a fraction of a second, or else a ventilator with minimal internal compliance and compressible volume must be devised. Heijman et al. used an ''insufflation catheter'', a small noncompliant lumen, to deliver a pulse of gas to the airway (Figure 1).[22] Sjostrand developed a prototype ventilator which delivers the inspiratory flow through a side-arm in a manner similar to that of a Sanders ventilating bronchoscope.[11] This airway attachment (Figure 2) was called the pneumatic valve. Initially, neither device incorporated an expiratory valve. Hence, they would be considered to be open systems. However, both designs attempted to limit or eliminate entrainment.

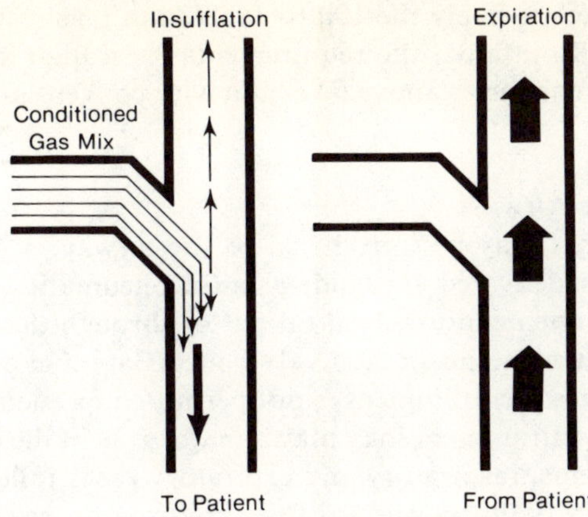

FIGURE 2. Schematic diagram of the "Pneumatic Valve" airway attachment. There is no expiratory valve. Entrainment is prevented by exhaust of gas during insufflation. A later modification included an expiratory valve to provide volume-controlled ventilation. (From Sjostrand, U., *Acta Anaesth. Scand.* Suppl., 64, 7, 1977. With permission.)

The insufflation catheter did not provide a low impedance source for entrainment gas. The pneumatic valve was designed to provide gas flow through the exhaust during inspiration. A later version of the side-arm, or pneumatic valve, also added an expiratory valve to enable delivery of volume-controlled. HFPPV.[13,23,24] In both of these devices, the inspiratory gas is derived from a high pressure source and periodically pulsed into the airway. Due to the low-volume, low-compressibility circuit the majority of the tidal volume is delivered in early inspiration with a decelerating flow pattern, and allows time for subsequent redistribution of gas in the lung. This is in contrast to the accelerating pattern of conventional ventilators.

A later variation of an HFPPV delivery system is described by Fletcher et al.[18] Gas flows from a pressure source, through a high resistance, to a valve near the proximal airway. Because the resistance in this circuit is much higher than that of the airway or breathing circuit, the flow source is assumed to have constant flow characteristics. Control of ventilation is provided by a rotary valve. The valve alternately opens the airway to the inspiratory and then the expiratory arm of the breathing circuit with a slight hold between each phase. This arrangement prevents both entrainment and the escape of gas during inspiration. It also provides for a slight inspiratory and expiratory pause, but can only provide a fixed I:E ratio. Chakrabarti and Sykes achieve a similar effect by the use of two valves, one for inspiration and one for expiration, operating off a common camshaft.[19] I:E ratio was 1:2 with a 15° inspiratory and expiratory pause. All of these designs keep compressible volume and ventilator compliance to a mimimum.

Because of the need for an almost instantaneous delivery of tidal volume, HFPPV ventilators must be able to deliver peak flows of 175 to 250 ℓ/min. This is beyond the capabilities of most conventional ventilators and circuits. The time-response of components, such as the expiratory valve, may be inadequate at higher rates. Also, the failure of limited-life components will be accelerated. Nonetheless, conventional ventilators have been employed to deliver HFPPV.[14-15,17,20] The Bennett MA-1B and MA-2 have been used in a self-triggering mode at maximum ventilation frequency and inspiratory flowrate. In this mode, a tidal volume of 70 to 90 mℓ at a rate of approximately 66 c/min can be expected. The I:E ratio will be approximately 0.3. The key to success in this approach is likely the 100 to 125 ℓ/min inspiratory flowrate these ventilators can produce. In infants, the requirements for a high inspiratory flowrate are not as extreme, and frequencies above 60 c/min with conventional ventilators are commonly used.[15,20,25,26]

2. Gas Delivery to the Airway

The inspiratory gases may be introduced to the airway in one of four ways with HFPPV. They may be delivered via a side-arm (or pneumatic valve),[23] an insufflation catheter,[22] a double-lumen endotracheal tube,[16] or through the main lumen of the endotracheal tube.[18] When the pneumatic valve, insufflation catheter, or double-lumen endotracheal tube is used, entrainment is not permitted or encouraged. This is in contrast to HFJV, where entrainment may play a major role in the efficacy of ventilation. In these HFPPV systems, inspiratory and expiratory gases follow different pathways. Initially, the expiratory pathway was left open. In order to provide volume-controlled ventilation, an expiratory valve was later added.[23,24] The rotary valve design of Fletcher et al.[18] uses the same airway lumen for inspiration and expiration, as do conventional ventilators when used for HFPPV, and their ventilator design inherently prevents entrainment or the escape of gas during inspiration. This is also true for the design of Chakrabarti and Sykes.[19]

Conventional ventilators with adult circuits are generally not suited to HFPPV because of the large internal ventilator and circuit compliance, large compressible volume, and significant dead space between the inspiratory and expiratory valves. With short inspiratory time, the gas flow must accelerate quickly, and volume losses to compliance and compression are more significant. Also, because the tidal volume is smaller, any volume losses or dead space volumes are a higher proportion of the available gas exchange volume. If a conventional ventilator is to be used for HFPPV, it is advisable to modify the circuit to eliminate as much volume and compliance as possible and locate the expiratory valve as close as practical to the airway.

3. Conditioning of Gases

Because of the high peak flow rates and rapid transitions from low to high flow, blending, heating, and humidifying of respiratory gas must receive special attention. A heater-humidifier place in the inspiratory path must introduce little resistance, compliance, or compressible volume. If gases are humidified prior to being supplied to the flow control valves, the flow-damping effects are eliminated; but now concerns arise about contamination and corrosion in the flow controller. It also must be assured that the peak flow demands of HFPPV do not exceed the capabilities of the oxygen blender and gas supply piping.

Minute volumes with HFPPV are greater than with CMV, even though tidal volumes are smaller. Because of this, total gas usage must be considered. It is conceivable that too many HFPPV devices in use simultaneously could quickly exhaust the hospital oxygen supply.

4. Monitoring and Safety

HFPPV generally involves the delivery of gases from a high pressure source at high flow rates. Hence, measuring and controlling airway pressure is of vital importance. Measurements should be obtained from the middle or distal airway to be assured that they are not affected by artifacts of high flow rates. The monitoring system must also be capable of accurate measurements at the higher frequencies employed with HFPPV. Generally, mechanical gauges are not adequate. When electronic transducers are used, in order to maintain lumen appropriate frequency response, attention must be given to the stiffness and lumen size of the measurement catheter. Although saline-filled catheters have been proposed, they may actually have worse frequency response characteristics than air-filled systems. It is desirable for the measuring system to have a frequency response several times higher than the ventilatory frequency in order to accurately record pressure transients. Catheter-tip transducers have superior response, but are costly. Alarms and safety features also should be provided on the ventilator to prevent over-pressurization of the airway.

Volume monitoring can be used in those devices which employ an expiratory valve. Ultrasonic flowmeters, specially designed pneumotachs, and hot-wire anemometers may be used.[24,27,28] Mechanical spirometers may introduce measurement errors due to their inertia and momentum which limit their time-response. Since gas flows are highly transient, it is common to collect or measure the total expired gas for a period and then divide by the frequency to infer a tidal volume. Volume monitoring is inaccurate in open systems because there is no way to confirm that all of the escaping gas has actually participated in exchange with the lung.

Respiratory gas analysis is also potentially useful with HFPPV. End-tidal measurements may be made if the response of the analyzer is adequate. However, it must be realized that the end-tidal gas may no longer represent alveolar concentrations. The reason for this is that the small tidal volume consists primarily of gas from the conducting airways.[29] Because of the small tidal volumes, gas analyzers with in-line sensors or low sample flow rates are indicated for end-tidal analysis. If ventilation can be momentarily interrupted, end-tidal analysis of the first full expiration may be used to estimate blood gas tensions.[30] Knowledge of the average concentration and total volume can be used to calculate the flux of the gas of interest.

As with conventional ventilation, monitoring for physiologic effect by arterial blood gas analysis is the best technique. Hemodynamic measurements are also indicated.

5. Operational Variables with HFPPV

Determinants of the effectiveness of gas exchange during HFPPV appear similar to conventional ventilation. Minute ventilation affects carbon dioxide removal; and MAP and inspired concentration affect oxygenation.[19,31-32] Beyond this, it is difficult to suggest settings for use of HFPPV in a particular system. The most commonly used HFPPV rate is 60 c/min (1 Hz). This rate is usually combined with an I:E ratio of 0.15 to 0.3. It is necessary to provide more time for expiration than for inspiration because expiration is passive and is governed by the mechanical time constants of the chest and airways. Peak airway pressures are generally lower with HFPPV than with conventional positive-pressure ventilation, presumably because of smaller tidal volumes. However, MAP is vary between being lower than those with CMV to being similar to or higher than those with CMV. End-expiratory pressures may be higher than with CMV. Some PEEP may be necessary to keep the lung above airway closure volume.[13] Most of the clinical experience with specifically designed HFPPV equipment is from endoscopies with open systems. Nomograms for total gas minute-flowrates to be used with specific devices have been developed, but estimates of required tidal volumes are not available.[13,33] Clinical experience with volume controlled devices, especially in patients with respiratory distress, is limited. Abu-Dbai et al.[14] achieved adequate ventilation with conventional ventilators delivering HFPPV with a tidal volume of 1 to 3 mℓ/kg at 66 to 70 c/min and an I:E ratio of 0.3. However, because of the varying compressible volumes and flow characteristics of different ventilator designs, it may not be possible to extrapolate these values to other systems.

C. HFJV

HFJV was first described by Klain and Smith in 1977 when they demonstrated that it was possible to provide adequate oxygen and carbon dioxide gas exchange using rapid pulsations of gas through a catheter inserted percutaneously into the trachea of dogs at ventilatory frequencies between 20 and 200 c/min.[34] Currently, HFJV generally refers to any method of ventilation by which an inspiratory pulse or jet of gas is delivered to the lungs through a small diameter catheter or orifice. Expiration is a passive process and depends upon the elastic recoil properties of the lungs and chest wall. A further characteristic inherent to HFJV is augmentation of the inspired volume delivered by the jet with additional gas entrained from the proximal airway. Inspiratory gas is entrained as long as a supplemental gas reservoir is provided. Clinically, ventilatory rates between 100 and 200 c/min are most common with HFJV. However, ventilatory frequencies as low as 50 c/min and as high as 1000 c/min have been used in some research protocols.

1. Methods of Generating and Controlling the Jet Pulse

Specific design details vary greatly among HFJV, especially since many of the devices described in research protocols are "one-of-a-kind" prototypes. However, all HFJV devices provide a method by which a high pressure gas source can be precisely interrupted to produce a controlled pulsed gas stream. Most devices utilize the 50 psi air and oxygen outlets found in most hospitals as the high pressure gas source, although they also can operate from compressed air and oxygen tanks. The inlet pressure to the ventilator, termed the driving pressure, can be adjusted with a standard pressure regulator. However, in commercially available HFJV ventilators, a means of regulating the driving pressure is incorporated into the device itself.

Control of the duration and the frequency of the jet pulse is usually accomplished by one of two methods. Fluidic control systems have been described by Smith et al.,[35] and Calkins et al.[36] These devices utilize a bistable fluid amplifier to initiate and terminate inspiration. An important advantage of fluidic controlled systems is their need for relatively few moving parts. This may be an important consideration if one considers the potential for fatigue and wear in a device that may function at a frequency in excess of 10 Hz for extended periods of time. More commonly however, control of the inspiratory pulse is accomplished by the use of an electronically controlled solenoid valve.[10,37] These systems are simple in design, but allow for independent control of both the duration and frequency of the inspiratory pulse. In some devices, the operation of the solenoid valve can be electronically coupled to the electrocardiogram, allowing for synchronization of the ventilator to any part of the QRS cycle.[37] A diagram of one such system is shown in Figure 3. It has been suggested that this might result in an augmentation of cardiac stroke volume.[38] Although it appears that this technique is of little cardiovascular benefit when myocardial function is normal, preliminary data suggest that syncyhronization of HFJV to the QRS cycle may enhance cardiac function when myocardial function is imparied.[39,40]

2. Gas Delivery to the Airway

Several techniques have been described for delivering the jet pulse to the airway. Ventilatory catheters are often placed proximally inside the lumen of an endotracheal tube (Figure 4).[41] Alternatively, the ventilating catheter can be placed in the distal trachea, either by a catheter attached externally to the endotracheal tube or via an extra lumen contained within the wall of the endotracheal tube itself (Figure 3).[4,36,39,42] Although adequate ventilation can be obtained irrespective of whether the ventilation catheter is in the proximal or distal airway, location of the ventilation catheter appears to be an important factor in determining the efficacy of ventilation. Calkins et al. have demonstrated in normal dogs that when frequency, inspiratory/expiratory ratio, and driving pressure were held constant, $PaCO_2$ varied linearly with catheter tip distance from the carina.[43] The mechanism underlying this observation is unclear. Greater ef-

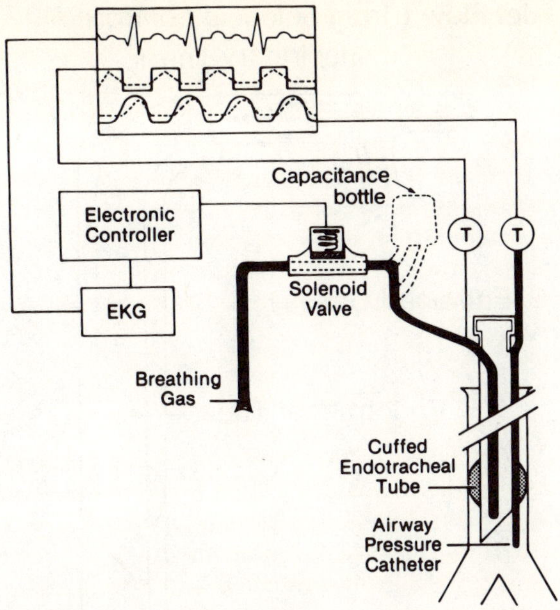

FIGURE 3. Schematic diagram of a HFJV system using a solenoid valve and delivery of the jet to the airway via a catheter to the distal endotracheal tube. The jet may alternatively be extruded in the wall of the endotracheal tube. The system shown uses an electronic controller to set the frequency and I:E ratio and allows synchronization of the jet pulse to a particular part of the heart's electrical cycle. (From Otto, C. W., Quan, S. F., Conahan, T. J., et al., *Anesth. Analg.*, 62, 298, 1983. With permission.)

ficiency of ventilation may simply be a result of bypassing tracheal deadspace. Alternatively, a distal jet location may enhance local gas mixing, thereby facilitating intrapulmonary gas transport. Bourby et al.[9] found that the same $PaCO_2$ was achieved with a smaller tidal volume with the distally located jet. The increase in jet injector volume necessary to achieve normocarbia was more than offset by a decrease in the amount of entrained gas, leading to a decrease in total tidal volume.

There may be disadvantages, however, to placement of the ventilation catheter distally in the trachea. In critically ill patients who are already intubated, re-intubation in order to place a distal catheter to deliver HFJV may place the patient at risk. In addition, the effects of distal vs. proximal jet placement on causing injury to the tracheal mucosa remain to be determined. Of more importance is that the amount of entrainment gas also differs between proximal and distal jet location. It has been shown that entrainment volume is significantly lower when the jet is placed distally compared with proximally.[4,9] The effect of jet location on entrainment volume is especially marked when the compliance of the respiratory system is quite low. In this clinical situation, for the same volume of gas delivered by the jet, pressure developed in the airways is greater than that observed when the respiratory system is more compliant. As pressure in the airway increases, the amount of entrainment volume falls, and may approach zero since the airway pressure gradient favoring entrainment is progressively reduced. This phenomenon is referred to as "stalling". Stalling appears to occur more frequently with distal as opposed to proximal jet delivery. If distal jet delivery is obtained by using a lumen incorporated within the wall of an endotracheal tube, less efficient entrainment may result. This is due in part, to the noncentral location of the jet deliv-

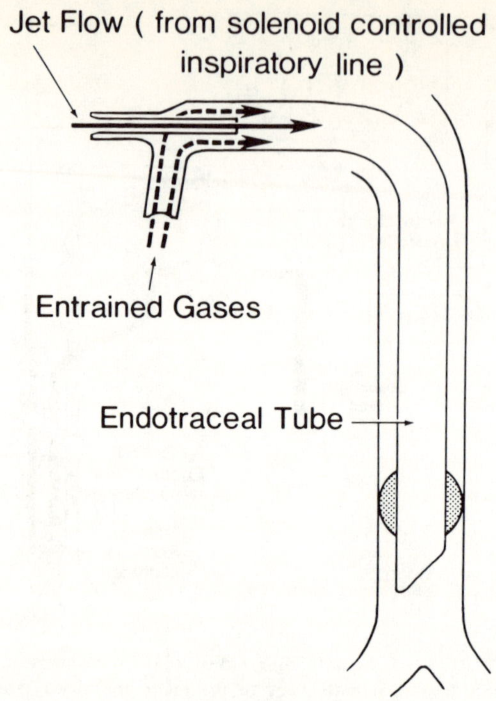

FIGURE 4. Schematic diagram of HFJV delivery to the airway using a proximal jet injector. Entrainment gases are provided from the breathing circuit through a side port in the swivel adapter. (Adapted from Carlon, G. C., Kahn, R. C., Howlan, W. S., et al., *Crit. Care Med.*, 9, 1, 1981. With permission.)

ery orifice (Coanda effect).[2] The efficiency of entrainment with regard to proximal or distal jet delivery is related also to endotracheal tube diameter. As endotracheal tube diameter decreases, airflow resistance related to the endotracheal tube increases. Therefore, even with proximal jet delivery, entrainment volume becomes insignificant with very small (i.e., 3.0 or 3.5 mm ID) endotracheal tubes. In such cases, since entrainment volume is of relatively little importance, distal jet delivery is more efficient. Hamilton et al. have studied entrainment with pediatric HFJV endotracheal tubes and concluded that entrainment efficiency can be affected by resistance in both the inlet tube and downstream airway, as well as proximity to the endotracheal tube opening.[44]

As originally described by Klain and Smith in dogs,[34] a jet ventilation catheter can be introduced percutaneously into the trachea. Although this technique has been proposed as being potentially useful during CPR,[45] disadvantages of introducing the jet pulse in this manner include the inability to monitor airway pressure during ventilation, and the possibility of inducing barotrauma if an obstruction to exhalation is present proximal to the end of the jet catheter.

Size of the ventilation catheter may also be an important factor in determining ventilatory efficacy. Carlon et al.[5] showed that entrained volume is higher with a 1.62 mm (14 G) catheter in comparison to a 1.06 mm (16 G) catheter. As expected, resistance was greater in the smaller catheter, resulting in higher reqired driving pressures. If mean airway pressures are comparable, however, the effects on gas exchange and cardiovascular function of 1.62 and 1.06 mm catheters are equivalent.[46] The ratio of the cross-sectional area of the ventilation catheter to the cross-sectional area of the tracheal airway may be a more important factor than the absolute size of the ventilation catheter itself. Calkins et al.[43] have demonstrated that lumen area ratios ranging from 1:6 to 1:11 are sufficient to insure normocarbia. If the cross-secitonal area of the catheter is larger than 1/6th the area of the expiratory lumen, incomplete expiration, gas trapping, and CO_2 retention may result.

3. Conditioning of Gases

During HFJV, there is movement of large volumes of gas at high flow rates into and out of the lungs. If nonhumidified gas is used, desiccation of the airway with inspissation of secretions, and possibly airway obstruction, may result. Kalin et al. showed impairment of mucociliary transport when humidifcation was inappropriate.[47] Inspired gases during HFJV are a mixture of entrained and pulsed gas. Although humidification of only the entrained gas is simple to do, adequate humidification is inlikely unless the pulsed gas is also humidified. Several methods of humidifying the pulsed gas have been described. In one system, water is infused in front of the jet at a slow constant rate, resulting in nebulization by the jet itself.[48] Another method involves slowly infusing water into the proximal end of the jet catheter.[49] Ramanathan et al. have described a coaxial catheter system in which water is entrained from an inner catheter by the negative pressure created by an outer jet delivery catheter.[50,51] Recently, Berman et al. demonstrated in an artificial lung model that directing the jet pulse through a modified heated wick-type humidifier delivered more humidity than a water infusion system.[52] Chatburn and McClellan describe a system which combines the infusion of water and a heated coil to provide 91% humidity gas at near body temperature.[53] Although it appears that adequate humidification can result from using any of the systems described, comparisons between systems in vivo have not yet been performed.

4. Monitoring and Safety

As with conventional positive pressure ventilators, HFJV requires monitoring and feedback systems so that safe and effective performance can be ensured. Although a number of variables can be monitored, such as inspired oxygen concentration and expired gas volumes, it is generally agreed that the most important monitoring variable during HFJV is airway pressure. The importance of monitoring airway pressure during HFJV is threefold. First, since HFJV is characterized by rapid pulsations of gas under high pressure and at high flow rates, dangerously high airway pressures can develop within a very short periods of time if there is an expiratory airway occlusion. An airway pressure monitoring system will allow for insertion of a rapid, automatic feedback loop to interrupt the jet before pulmonary barotrauma can develop. Second, an airway pressure monitoring system can be used as a sensor to detect hazardous low pressure situations, such as accidental disconnection or jet malfunction. Third, airway pressure appears to correlate with the efficiency of gas exchange during HFJV, and is one of the control variables that can be adjusted to optimize gas exchange.[54]

When monitoring airway pressure during HFJV, the location of the monitoring port is an important factor in determining the accuracy of the pressure measurements. As demonstrated recently by Waterson et al.,[54] airway pressures measured at or above the jet are misleadingly low. However, the optimum distance below the jet for accurate pressure measurements is still uncertain.

The use of gas analysis with HFJV is even more difficult than with HFPPV. Not only are the ventilatory frequencies higher, but the mixing of gases due to entrainment and stalling make it hard to obtain a representative expiratory sample. The situation is further complicated by the open nature of the system. The technique of interrupting ventilation momentarily and capturing the first end-tidal value is useful in the absence of gas analyzers with fast enough response for breath-by-breath determinations during HJFV.[30,55,56]

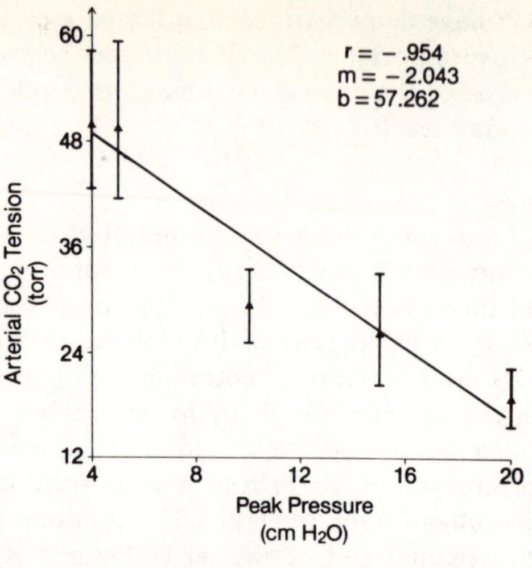

FIGURE 5. Relationship between arterial carbon dioxide tension and peak airway pressure with HFJV at 150 c/min and 30% inspiratory time. (From Calkins, J. M., Waterson, C. K., Quan, S. F., et al., in *Perspectives in High Frequency Ventilation*, Scheck, P. A., Sjostrand, U. H., Smith, R. B., Eds., Martinus Nijhoff, Boston, 1983. With permission.)

Volume measurements are also more difficult with HFJV. Attempts have been made to collect total expired gas and hence to compute a minute or tidal volume.[5] This technique, however, neglects the possibility of stalling and disregards the open nature of the system which allows escape of gas during inspiration which has not particpiated in gas exchange within the lung. The optimum flow or volume measurement system should be able to simultaneously and separately measure jet and entrainment flow. Any exhaust flow measured while the jet was still on would be subtracted from the tidal volume total. Although such a total system has not yet been devised, Watt et al.[57] used a pitot tube to measure the highly transient jet gas flows. Special consideration must be given to flow measuring devices to be used with the jet because of the high flow rates and rapid changes in gas flows. Devices to be used to measure entrainment gas must be capable of determining the direction of flow and should not add significant impedance to flow, since any added resistance will impede both entrainment and exhaust.

5. Operational Characteristics

Determinants of gas exchange during HFJV are different than those during CMV. With CMV, if CO_2 production and dead space remain constant, carbon dioxide gas exchange is determined by the combination of ventilatory frequency and tidal volume. In contrast, the important variables influencing CO_2 gas exchange during HFJV appear to be airway pressure (Paw); I:E ratio, re-expressed as percent inspiratory time (I%); frequency; and jet flow waveshape. As expected, peak airway pressures, measured in the distal airway, are lower with HFJV than with CMV. However, mean and end-expiratory pressures are dependent on several ventilation parameters and may be higher, lower, or the same as with CMV.

Efficiency of CO_2 elimination during HFJV appears to be directly related to increasing airway pressure. In studies performed by Calkins et al.[43] and Waterson et al.[54] in normal dogs, $PaCO_2$ was observed to be inversely correlated with both peak airway pressure (Figure 5) and the excursion between peak and end-expiratory pressure,

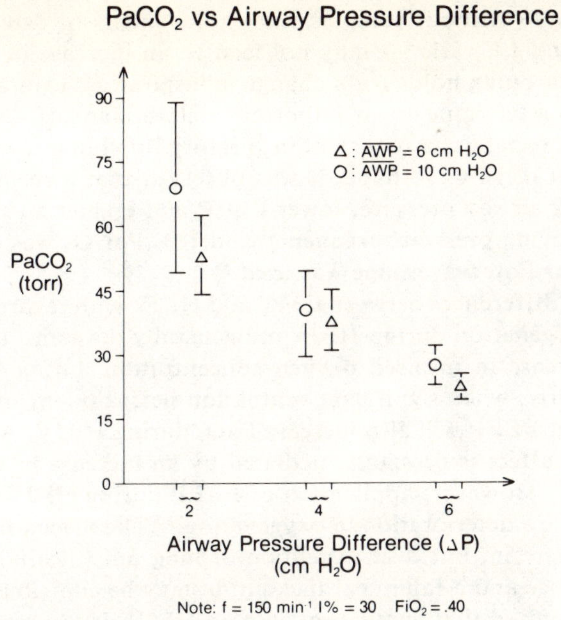

FIGURE 6. Relationship between arterial carbon dioxide tension and airway pressure difference (ΔP = peak — end-expiratory pressure) at mean airway pressures of 6 and 10 cm H_2O, 150 c/min, and 30% inspiratory time. (From Waterson, C. K., Militzer, H. W., Quan, S. F., and Calkins, J. M., *Crit. Care Med.*, 12, 742, 1984. With permission.)

termed airway pressure difference (Figure 6). Rouby et al.,[58] Calkins et al.,[43] and Waterson et al.[54] have also shown that CO_2 elimination improves with increasing AWP. However, airway pressure excursion appears to a better indicator of gas exchange than does either peak or AWP.[54] Airway pressure is primarily a function of the driving pressure. As driving pressure increases, so does Paw. However, because of variability in the resistance of jet delivery devices and in the respiratory system mechanics among patients, there is no consistent relationship between drive pressure and the resultant airway pressure. Thus, the prediction of physiologic effect from a given driving pressure is not reliable. Additional factors which affect a Paw are I%, frequency, and expiratory resistance. Manipulation of driving pressure, I%, frequency, and expiratory resistance allow for adjustment of peak and mean airway pressures.

If frequency and airway pressure excursion are held constant, $PaCO_2$ varies directly with an increase in inspiratory/expiratory ratio (I:E) or percent inspiratory time (I%).[43] It is presumed that this effect is related to an inadequate amount of time for expiration, which leads to impaired gas exchange. Similarly, between frequencies of 200 and 900 c/min in both dogs and humans, an increase in ventilatory frequency results in a higher $PaCO_2$.[43] This phenomenon also may be caused by the lack of expiratory time. Expiratory flow rate is determined by the time constants of the lung. Hence, if more gas is put in than can be expelled during the expiratory phase, there will be an increase in lung pressure and volume as the lung increases the driving force for expiration. If peak airway pressure is maintained constant, it is observed that end-tidal pressure also increases and the excurison pressure decreases. This increase in end-tidal pressure at high frequencies and high I:E ratios, due to incomplete expiration, has been termed "auto-PEEP". It can be seen, therefore, that an increase in ventilatory frequency only — without compensatory adjustments of driving pressure, expiratory resistance, and I:E ratio — may not lead to an increase in gas exchange efficiency. The same reasoning holds for a change in inspiratory/expiratory ratio.

Finally, jet flow waveshape is an important determinant of CO_2 elimination. In studies comparing a rectangular (constant inspiratory flow) to a sawtooth (accelerating inspiratory flow) jet drive waveshape, it was observed that a rectangular shape produced a higher peak airway pressure, lower PEEP and greater airway pressure excursion at the same driving pressure, frequency and I%. $PaCO_2$ was significantly lower when the rectangular flow waveshape was used.[59]

In contrast to the differences between CMV and HFJV with regard to CO_2 exchange, determinants of oxygenation during HFJV are generally the same as during CMV. As with CMV, an increase in inspired oxygen concentration during HFJV results in a higher PaO_2. Similarly, when significant ventilation-perfusion mismatching is present, elevation of AWP or PEEP will also increase PaO_2 during HFJV. As demonstrated by Rouby et al.,[58] this effect is probably mediated by an increase in functional residual capacity with HFJV. However, application of PEEP during HFJV when lung disease is minimal may cause a deterioration in oxygenation.[60] The mechanism underlying this observation is not certain, but over-distention of lung units leading to an increase in physiologic dead space and a fall in cardiac output may be contributing factors.

It should be recognized that ventilation with an HFJV device represents an interaction between the properties of the gas imparted by the ventilator and the mechanics of the respiratory system. In this respect a HFJV device behaves quite similarly to a pressure limited, positive-pressure ventilator. For the same ventilator settings, marked alterations in gas delivery to the patient can occur if there are changes in respiratory system mechanics. Therefore, standard ventilator settings with HFJV that would lead to satisfactory gas exchange in most patients are more difficult to derive than with CMV. Nevertheless, it appears that a frequency of 150 c/min, I% of 30%, and an airway pressure excursion between 5 and 10 cm H_2O will result in adequate gas exchange in patients with relatively normal lungs.

6. Design Features of a Clinical HFJV Device

All HFJV devices should provide means for independent control of driving pressure, I:E ratio, and frequency. A PEEP control is also desirable but not absolutely necessary since an external PEEP device can be placed on the exhalation limb of the patient's ventilator circuit. An airway pressure monitoring system with an automatic feedback to terminate jet pulses if over pressurization occurs is an absolute requirement. Alarms for low pressure, disconnection, or jet malfunction also should be present. Desirable features include; (1) a demand or constant flow reservoir system to provide entrainment gas; (2) an air-oxygen blender intrinsic to the ventilator; and (3) digital monitors of peak, mean, and end-expiratory airway pressures, as well as the airway pressure excursion between peak and end-expiratory pressure.

D. HFOV

The term HFOV refers to a technique which has little in common with either conventional ventilation or the previously discussed techniques of HFPPV and HFJV. HFOV involves the use of a pump, or driver, to alternately compress and decompress the gas column in the airway while moving tidal volumes much less than the anatomical dead space. It is generally used at much higher frequencies than HFPPV or HFJV, in the range of 900 c/min, but has been reported as low as 60 c/min (1 Hz) and as high as 2400 c/min (40 Hz). Although first described by Lunkenheimer in 1972 as a means of enhancing gas exchange during apneic oxygenation,[61,62] the principles involved were recognized much earlier.[63,64] A device to "vibrate the airways" was patented in 1959.[65]

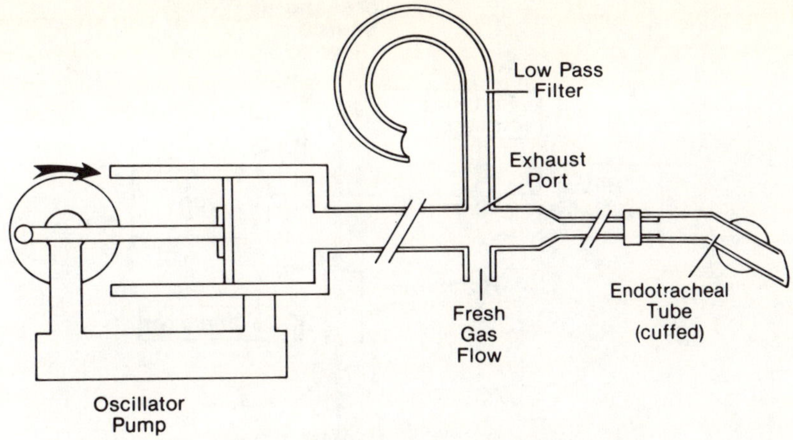

FIGURE 7. Schematic diagram of an open design HFOV system. The "low pass filter" allows for the escape of steady bias flow while presenting impedance to high-frequency oscillations. (From Butler, W. J., Bohn, D. J., Bryan, A. C., and Froese, A. B., *Anesth. Analg.*, 59, 577, 1980. With permission.)

More recently, much attention has been given to HFOV as a means of ventilating a patient's lungs without the cyclical lung inflation and deflation inherent in the other techniques. There is also considerable interest in respiratory gas transport mechanisms during HFOV since its effectiveness seems to be somewhat independent of lung mechanics. If so, it could potentially be useful for patients with impaired lung mechanics — particularly for those with nonhomogenous time constants within the lung. There seem to be two important reasons why HFOV is independent of lung mechanics. First, it operates well above the resonant frequency of the lung and beyond the time constants of most airway units. Second, it has an active expiratory phase during which it draws out of the airway the same amount of gases it puts in during inspiration.

1. Equipment for Delivery of HFOV

At first glance, the delivery systems for HFOV appear quite simple and straightforward. A pump or driver system is used to produce the pressure oscillations. The pump may be either a piston or diaphram type, and the drivers are often one or more large loudspeakers. However, the volumes of gas to be moved at such high frequencies place quite a load on the pump or driver. Also, internal compressible volume and compliance must be minimized to avoid losing the whole stroke volume to compression of gas within the device. Because of simplicity, the majority of HFOV oscillators produce sinusoidal waveshapes with an I:E ratio of 1:1, but there is no evidence that this is optimum for gas exchange.

There are various means for providing fresh gas and accommodating the exhaust of expired gas in HFOV ventilators. Bohn et al.[66,67] designed an open system which used a length of coiled tubing for the exhaust path. The length and diameter of this tubing was chosen to present a high impedance to the oscillatory flow, while providing only a minimal resistance to steady flow. Fresh gas was introduced to the proximal airway. This system is shown in Figure 7. Slutsky et al.[68,69] devised a closed system by the introduction of high impedance valves in both the inlet and outlet for the bias flow as shown in Figure 8. The fresh gas was supplied from a pressure source and exhausted to a vacuum through valves so that none of the oscillation volume would be lost. While this makes accurate measurements of gas compositions and volumes possible, it prevents spontaneous breathing. Ngeow and Mitzner[70] developed a system to allow the

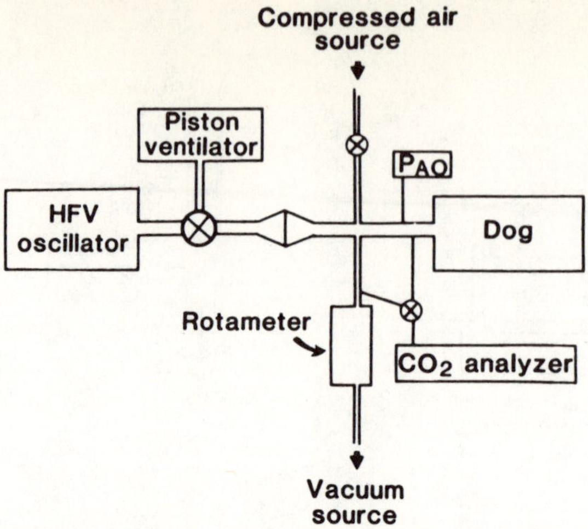

FIGURE 8. Schematic diagram of a closed design HFOV system. The fresh bias flow is provided from a compressed gas source through a restriction valve and exhausts to vacuum through another resistance. This design facilitates gas flux measurement. (From Slutsky, A. S., Drazen, J. M., Ingram, R. H., et al., *Science*, 209, 609, 1980. Copyright 1980. With permission.)

recirculation of gases in the HFOV circuit by incorporating a recirculator pump, Sodalime absorber, and heat exchanger. Boynton et al.[71] report the use of the Emerson Airway Vibrator[65] in combination with the conventional BABYbird Infant Ventilator (Bird-3M, St. Paul, Minn.). The infant ventilator provides the conditioned fresh gas flow and periodic IMV tidal volumes.

2. Gas Delivery to the Airway

HFOV generally uses a standard endotracheal tube. The oscillatory flow is directed through the main lumen of the tube and the bias flow is introduced via cross connector to the proximal airway. However, Rossing et al. experimented with using an extra lumen in the endotracheal tube to introduce fresh gas in the distal airway, and found that carbon dioxide removal was 50% more effective than when the bias flow was in the proximal airway.[72] This finding is consistent with the hypothesis that the majority of the resistance to gas transport by HFOV is in the endotracheal tube. This is presumed to be due to the role of augmented or enhanced gas dispersion as the primary gas transport phenomena with HFOV, as opposed to the major role of bulk flow with conventional ventilation. Hence, any increase in diffusion path length would impede gas exchange; and any decrease in length, such as moving the fresh gas introduction site to the distal airway, would enhance gas transport. The flow resistance of the endotracheal tube must also be taken into account at such high frequencies. Substantial pressure gradients can be generated due to high flow rates.

3. Conditioning of Gases

The warming and humidification of gases for HFOV is easier than it is with either HFPPV or HFJV. Since the bias flow is a steady stream, the conditioning equipment need not accommodate the rapid flow-transients observed with other HFV techniques. Also, the volume and compliance of the humidifier is not seen by the HFOV circuit because of the high impedance of the bias flow input valve. Furthermore, the fresh gas flow rate is much lower ($\ll$ 100 ℓ/min) and well within the capabilities of normal gas mixers and humidifiers.

4. Monitoring and Safety

As with other HVF techniques, the primary variable of interest is airway pressure. Because of the pressure gradients in the airways, it is important to consider the location of the monitor. The pressure in the peripheral airways may be different than pressures in the central airways.[73,74] The relationship of airway pressure to gas exchange is not as apparent with HFOV, but the potential for barotrauma or cardiovascular depression due to over pressurization still exists. Such a situation could easily occur if the exhaust for bias flow is occluded. Clinical devices require a continuous measure of airway pressure, and a means of relieving circuit pressure and interrupting oscillation in the event of over-pressurization.

End-tidal gas analysis is not possible. However, measures of carbon dioxide flux can be made by analyzing the average concentration in the exhausting bias flow. To provide maximum accuracy, a closed system is preferable,[68-72,75] but this technique can also be used with an open system if the low-pass filter is long enough to prevent mixing with room air.

Lung volumes are also of more interest with HFOV. Since the technique involves very little cyclic expansion of the lung, it is presumed that it is necessary to maintain the lung above its FRC, or the airway's closing volume, if there has been a decrease in FRC due to lung pathology.[69,76] Use of a sigh manuever and CPAP is necessary to maintain oxygenation. It is hypopthesized that the sigh opens the collapsed airways and recruits additional gas exchanging lung units. The CPAP is used to keep the recruited lung units open. It is assumed that pressure measured in the distal trachea reflects the expansion or recoil forces of the central conducting airways. It also is assumed that pressure gradients exist between the central and peripheral airways. Since positive pressure in the peripheral airways would cause them to expand, perhaps lung volumes can be used to infer pressures in the peripheral airways. Because it is desired to obtain a mean or pseudo-static lung volume, the use of magnetometers or plethysmographic techniques which can register static volume changes is indicated.

5. Operational Variables

HFOV systems usually provide independent control of oscillation frequency, volume of oscillation (amplitude or stroke volume), bias or fresh gas flow rate, and expiratory resistance or AWP. In an attempt to identify the variables affecting carbon dioxide gas exchange with HFOV, Slutsky et al.[69,75] studied the effects of frequency, amplitude, and lung volume. Their results indicated that gas exchange efficiency is most strongly related to the product of amplitude and frequency. This is not surprising, since this product is analagous to minute ventilation, except that the volume of oscillation was always less than the total estimated anatomic and equipment dead space. At lung volumes above FRC, there was no effect of lung volume on carbon dioxide flux rate. Bohn et al.[66] suggested that there is an optimum oscillatory frequency. In their experiments on dogs, this was found to be 900 c/min (15 Hz). However, due to the frequency dependence of the open-design exhaust system, it is questionable whether the tidal volume delivered to the airway was constant at all frequencies. Other investigators have been able to achieve normocarbia with frequencies over the range of 120 to 2400 c/min (2 to 40 Hz). The situation with stroke volumes is more confusing. Butler et al[67] used tidal volumes of between 50 and 150 mℓ in adult humans at 900 c/min (15 Hz) with body weights between 34 and 100 kg. This is approximately 1.5 mℓ/kg. However, in dogs a more typical figure is 3 mℓ/kg.[66,69]

The effects of bias flow on gas exchange have not been independently studied. However, from comparing the results of Bohn et al.[66] to that of Suwa and Tagami,[77] it appears that increasing the bias flow increases gas exchange. This is also supported by the work of Rossing et al.,[72] studying the effect of fresh gas flow placement. It appears that higher bias flows or placing the fresh gas flow optimally in the airway helps to wash expired gas out of the system. Bias gas in-flow rate or expiratory resistance can also be used to control AWP. This in turn influences lung volume.

E. HFBSO

As alternatives to conventional positive-pressure ventilation have been developed, there has also been interest in ways of providing ventilation without connection to the airway. The Emerson Wrap-Around Ventilator,[78] Cuirass ventilator,[79] and Iron Lung attempted to mimic spontaneous ventilation by surrounding the thorax or body with a fluctuating negative (subatmospheric) pressure. While successful in many cases, there are some situations in which they fail. Furthermore, they are always difficult to use, with nursing care difficult to provide and patient acceptance less than enthusiastic. More recently, however, there have been attempts to provide ventilation by applying high frequency pressure pulses to the chest or pleural surface.

In high frequency externally applied ventilation, pressure oscillations are applied either to the air in a chamber surrounding the subject (HFBSO)[80,81] or to the surface of the chest or lung itself (HFCWO).[82,83] In the former case, a momentary pressure differential is created between the airways and atmosphere. This pressure difference is caused by phase lag and propogation time down the airways. When the oscillations are directly applied to the body, expiration is usually active and inspiration occurs due to passive recoil. It is possible, however, for the oscillation pressure around the body to be negative, thereby permitting active inspiration and passive expiration, as described by Chang in this book.

Although it has been shown that HFBSO can provide ventilatory support on some cases, it is still only in its early experimental stages, Nevertheless, ventilation without connection to the airway is intriguing. At this time, many questions need answers. For instance, can it be used when FRC is reduced below closing capacity? What are its hemodynamic effects? When is it effective, and when is it not? These questions and others require further investigation.

III. HFV REGULATORY STATUS

Before any new medical device can be marketed in the U.S., it must go through an approval process with the Food and Drug Administration's (FDA) Bureau of Medical Devices. For life support devices, such as ventilators, one of two processes (termed the 510K process or the PMA process) is usually followed.[84-86] These processes are described below in simplified form.

If it is a totally new technique, Pre-Market Approval (PMA) is required. Data must be acquired to show its safety and efficacy. An Investigational Device Exemption (IDE) from the FDA is necessary to allow the gathering of these data. Under the provisions of the IDE, clinical trials may be conducted to prove that the device works in the way it is claimed without undue risk to the patient, and that labeling, instructions, and manufacturing methods are adequate. The data gathered under the IDE is then presented to the FDA and a PMA may be granted to allow the sale and distribution of the device. Alternatively, the PMA may not be granted and more data may be requested.

If a device is substantially equivalent to one which was on the market in the U.S. prior to May 28, 1976, the manufacturer can apply for a 510 K approval. In support of this application, data must show that the device is functionally the same as the pre-1976 device. There is some interpretation of what constitutes substantial or functional eqivalence. If approval is granted, the device can be sold and distributed, but only for those uses approved under the 510 K for which the pre-1976 device was sold.

As of January, 1985, only three HFV systems have been approved for sale in the U.S. (others are available in Europe). All three are HFJV devices and are limited to a maximum frequency of 150 c/min. There have been two approved for use in laryngoscopies, bronchoscopies, and bronchopleural fistulaes (Model 300 and Model 303, Healthdyne, Marietta, GA). One is approved only for laryngoscopies and bronchoscopies (Model VS600, Instrument Development Corp., Pittsburgh, PA).

IV. SUMMARY

A host of systems have been proposed to deliver HFV. Each system has advantages and disadvantages which merit consideration. However, there are certain concerns which apply to all HFV delivery systems. First, they should be safe. Many of the experimental devices do not provide adequate monitoring and safety systems for unattended routine clinical use. Second, rules for manipulating operational variables need to be developed so the devices can be used by less experienced users in new situations. Third, designs need to be adapted for clinical use. Design factors such as ease of use, reliability, and failsafe modes should be considered. Fourth, the issue of gas consumption needs to be addressed. An ICU full of HFJV devices could quickly exhaust the hospital's oxygen supply. Fifth, adequate humidification and warming systems are needed, particularly with HFJV. And finally, a rationale for the application of HFV needs to be developed. As more data become available, it will be easier to decide in which situation HFV is indicated and which technique (HFPPV, HFJV, HFOV) is appropriate, or to conclude that HFV might be contraindicated for a specific patient.

REFERENCES

1. Froese, A. B., *High frequency ventilation: a critical assessment,* in *Critical Care: State of the Art,* Vol. 5., Society of Critical Care Medicine, Fullerton, Calif., 1984, 1.
2. Markland, E. and Boucher, R. F., Fundamentals of fluidics, in *A Guide to Fluidics,* Conway, A., Ed., Macdonald and Co., London, 1971.
3. Miodownik, S., Ray, C., Carlon, G., et al., High frequency jet ventilation: technical implications, *Crit. Care Med.,* 12, 718, 1984.
4. Davey, A. J., Lay, G. R., and Leigh, J. M., High frequency venturi jet ventilation, *Anaesthesia,* 37, 947, 1982.
5. Carlon, G. C., Ray, C., Griffin, J., et al., Tidal volume and airway pressure on high frequency jet ventilation, *Crit. Care Med.,* 11, 83, 1983.
6. Carlon, G. C. and Howland, W. S., Clinical experience with high frequency jet ventilation, in *International Anesthesiology Clinics,* Vol. 21, Smith, R. B. and Sjstrand, U. H., Eds., Little, Brown, Boston, 1983.
7. Rouby, J. J., Ecoffey, C., Benhamou, D., et al., High-frequency jet ventilation: effects of changing the internal diameter of the injector cannula, *Anesthesiology,* 61 A521, 1984.
8. Rouby, J. J., Benhamou, D., Simonneau, G., et al., Factors influencing tidal volume during high-frequency jet ventilation, *Anesthesiology,* 61, A505, 1984.
9. Rouby, J. J., Benhamou, D., Ecoffey, C., et al., High-frequency jet ventilation: a comparative study of proximal and distal injection, *Anesthesiology,* 61 A506, 1984.
10. Carlon, G. C., Miodownik, S., Ray, C., et al., Technical aspects and clinical implications of high frequency jet ventilation with a solenoid valve, *Crit. Care Med.,* 9, 47, 1981.
11. Sjostrand, U., Review of the physiological rationale for and development of high-frequency positive pressure ventilation — HFPPV, *Acta Anaesth. Scand.,* 64, 7, 1977.
12. Jonzon, A., Oberg, P. A., Sedin, G., et al., High frequency positive-pressure ventilation by endotracheal insufflation, *Acta Anaesth. Scan.,* Suppl. 43, 1, 1971.
13. Sjostrand, U. H., High-frequency positive-pressure ventilation (HFPPV): a review, *Crit. Care Med.,* 8, 345, 1980.

14. Abu-Dbai, J., Flatau, E., Lev, A., et al., The use of conventional ventilators for high frequency positive pressure ventilation, *Crit. Care Med.*, 11, 356, 1983.
15. Bland, R. D., Kim, M. H., Light, M. J., et al., High frequency mechanical ventilation in severe hyaline membrane disease: an alternative treatment?, *Crit. Care Med.*, 8, 275, 1980.
16. Babinski, M. F. and Smith, R. B., High frequency positive pressure ventilation for abdominal surgery, *Anesth. Analg.*, 63, 182, 1984.
17. Pinchak, A. C., Hagen, J. F., Hancock, D., et al., High-frequency positive-pressure ventilation with the MA-1 ventilator, *Crit. Care Med.*, 12, 810, 1984.
18. Fletcher, P. R., Epstein, M. A., and Epstein, R. A., A new ventilator for physiologic studies during high-frequency ventilation, *Respir. Physiol.*, 47, 21, 1982.
19. Chakrabarti, M. K. and Sykes, M. K., Cardiorespiratory effects of high frequency intermittent positive pressure ventilation in the dog, *Br. J. Anaesth.*, 52, 475, 1980.
20. Wren, W. S., High frequency positive pressure ventilation (HFPPV) in a newborn infant with ruptured lungs, *Br. J. Anaesth.*, 55, 575, 1983.
21. Fletcher, P. R. and Epstein, R. A., Constancy of physiological dead space during high-frequency ventilation, *Respir. Physiol.*, 47, 39, 1982.
22. Heijman, K., Heijman, L., Jonzon, A., et al., High frequency positive pressure ventilation during anaesthesia and routine surgery in man, *Acta Anaesth. Scand.*, 16, 176, 1972.
23. Sjstrand, U., Pneumatic systems facilitating treatment of respiratory insufficiency with alternative use of IPPV/PEEP, HFPPV/PEEP, CPPB, or CPAP, *Acta Anaesth. Scand.*, Suppl. 64, 123, 1977.
24. Wattwil, M., Sjostrand, U. H., and Borg, U. R., Comparative studies of IPPV and HFPPV with PEEP in critical care patients I: a clinical evaluation, *Crit. Care Med.*, 11, 30, 1983.
25. Bland, R. D. and Sedin, E. G., High frequency mechanical ventilation in the treatment of neonatal respiratory distress, in *International Anesthesiology Clinics*, Vol. 21, Smith, R. B. and Sjstrand, U. H., Eds., Little, Brown, Boston, 1983.
26. Eyal, F. G., Arad, I. D., Godder, K., et al., High-frequency positive-pressure ventilation in neonates, *Crit. Care Med.*, 12, 793, 1984.
27. Bertram, C. D., Flowmeter for high frequency ventilation on the pneumotach principle, *Aust. Phys. Eng. Sci. Med.*, 7, 85, 1984.
28. Hancock, D. E., Pinchak, A. C., and Hagen, J. F., Flow-monitoring system for high-frequency ventilation, *Crit. Care Med.*, 12, 824, 1984.
29. Rolly, G. and Versichelen, L., Gasanalysis by massspectrometry during high frequency ventilation, in *Perspectives in High Frequency Ventilation*, Scheck, P. A., Sjstrand, U. H., and Smith, R. B., Eds., Martinus Nijhoff, Boston, 1983.
30. Mihm, F. G., Feeley, T. W., Rodarte, A., et al., Monitoring high frequency jet ventilation by end-tidal carbon dioxide concentrations, *Anesthesiology*, 57, A87, 1982.
31. Wattwil, L. M., Sjstrand, U. H., Borg, U. R., et al., Comparative studies of CPPV and HFPPV with PEEP in critical care patients II: studies on intrapulmonary gas distribution, *Crit. Care Med.*, 11, 38, 1983.
32. Smith, R. B., Sjstrand, U. H., and Babinski, M. F., Technical considerations using high frequency positive pressure ventilation and high frequency jet ventilation, in *International Anesthesiology Clinics*, Vol 21, Smith, R. B. and Sjstrand, U. H., Eds., Little, Brown, Boston, 1983.
33. Borg, U., Eriksson, I., and Sjostrand, U., High-frequency positive-pressure ventilation (HFPPV): a review based upon its use during bronchoscopy and for laryungoscopy and microlaryngeal surgery under general anesthesia, *Anesth. Analg.*, 59, 594, 1980.
34. Klain, M. and Smith, R. B., High frequency percutaneous transtracheal jet ventilation, *Crit. Care Med.*, 5, 280, 1977.
35. Smith, R. B., Klain, M., Babinski, M. F., Limits of high frequency percutaneous transtracheal jet ventilation using a fluidic logic controlled ventilator, *Can. Anaesth. Soc. J.*, 27, 351, 1980.
36. Calkins, M. J., Waterson, C. K., Hameroff, S. R., et al., A simple flueric high frequency jet ventilator, *Anesth. Analg.*, 61, 138, 1982.
37. Calkins, J. M., Waterson, C. K., Hameroff, S. R., et al., Jet pulse characteristics for high frequency jet ventilation in dogs, *Anesth. Analg.*, 61, 293, 1982.
38. Klain, M. and Keszler, H., Circulation assist by high frequency ventilation, *Crit. Care Med.*, 7, 232, 1980.
39. Otto, C. W., Quan, S. F., Conahan, T. J., et al., Hemodynamic effects of high frequency jet ventilation, *Anesth. Analg.*, 62, 298, 1983.
40. Pinsky, M. R., Matuschak, G., Birnardi, L., et al., Hemodynamic effect of cardiac cycle specific increases in intrathoracic pressure, *Am. Rev. Respir. Dis.*, 129, A99, 1984.
41. Carlon, G. C., Kahn, R. C., Howland, W. S., et al., Clinical experience with high frequency jet ventilation, *Crit. Care Med.*, 9, 1, 1981.

42. Babinski, M. F., Bunegin, L., Smith, R. B., et al., Application of double lumen trachel tubes for HFV, *Anesthesiology,* 55, A370, 1981.
43. Calkins, J. M., Waterson, C. K., Quan, S. F., et al., Effects of high frequency jet ventilation design and operational variables upon arterial blood gas tensions, in *Perspectives in High Frequency Ventilation,* Scheck, P. A., Sjostrand, U. H., and Smith, R. B., Eds., Martinus Nijhoff, Boston, 1983.
44. Hamilton, L. H., Londino, J. M., Linehan, J. H., et al., Pediatric endotracheal tube designed for high-frequency ventilation, *Crit. Care Med.,* 12, 988, 1984.
45. Brader, E., Klain, M., Safer, P., et al., High frequency jet ventilation versus IPPV in cardiopulmonary resuscitation for asphyxia in dogs, *Crit. Care Med.,* 9, 162, 1981.
46. Bluth, L., Banner, M., and Gallagher, T. J., HFPPV: physiologic effect of injector size, *Anesthesiology,* 53, S403, 1980.
47. Klain, M., Nordin, U., and Keszler, H., Mucociliary transport with and without humidification in high frequency ventilation, *Anesthesiology,* 57, A86, 1982.
48. Turnbull, A. D., Carlon, G., Howland, W. S., et al., High frequency jet ventilation in major airway or pulmonary disruption, *Ann. Thrac. Surg.,* 32, 468, 1981.
49. Schuster, D. P., Klain, M., and Snyder, J. V., Comparison of high frequency jet ventilation to conventional ventilation during severe acute respiratory failure in humans, *Crit. Care Med.,* 10, 625, 1982.
50. Ramanathan, S., Arismendy, J., Gandhi, S., et al., A new jet ventilation catheter, *Anesthesiology,* 57, A169, 1982.
51. Ramanathan, S., Arismendy, J., Gandhi, S., et al., Coaxial catheter for hidification during jet ventilation, *Anesth. Analg.,* 61, 689, 1982.
52. Berman, L. S., Herad, S. O., and Banner, M. J., Humidification techniques for high frequency jet ventilation, *Crit. Care Med.,* 12, 284, 1984.
53. Chatburn, R. L. and McClellan, L. D., A heat and humidification system for high frequency jet ventilation, *Respir. Care,* 27, 1386, 1982.
54. Waterson, C. K., Militzer, H. W., Quan, S. F., et al., Airway pressure as a measure of gas exchange during high frequency jet ventilation, *Crit. Care Med.,* 12, 742, 1984.
55. Lobo, D. P., Brauer, F. S., Ciobanu, M., et al., Monitoring high frequency jet ventilation during anesthesia, *Anesthesiology,* 61, A171, 1984.
56. Mihm, F. G., Feeley, T. W., and Rodarte, A., Monitoring end-tidal carbon dioxide tensions with high frequency jet ventilation in dogs with normal lungs, *Crit. Care Med.,* 12, 180, 1984.
57. Watt, R. C., Waterson, C. K., and Calkins, J. M., Computer analysis of flow transient effects in high frequency jet ventilation, *Proc. AAMI 18th Annu. Meet.,* 131, 1983.
58. Rouby, J. J., Fusciardi, J., Bourgain, J. L., et al., High frequency jet ventilation in post-operative respiratory failure: determinants of oxygenation, *Anesthesiology,* 59, 281, 1983.
59. Calkins, J. M., Waterson, C. K., Hameroff, S. R., et al., Jet pulse characteristics for high frequency jet ventilation in dogs, *Anesth. Analg.,* 61, 293, 1982.
60. Calkins, J. M., Waterson, C. K., Quan, S. F., et al., Operational guidelines for high frequency jet ventilation, Unpublished.
61. Lunkenheimer, P. P., Rafflenbeul, W., Keller, H., et al., Application of transtracheal pressure oscillations as modification of "Diffusion Respiration", *Br. J. Anaesth.,* 44, 627, 1972.
62. Noack, F. W., Lunkenheimer, P. P., Ising, H., et al., Light- and electron microscopic investigation of pulmonary tissue after high-frequency positive-pressure ventilation (HFPPV), *Anaesthesist,* 24, 171, 1975.
63. Taylor, G. I., Dispersion of soluble matter in solvent flowing slowly through a tube, *Proc. R. Soc. London. Ser. A,* 219, 186, 1953.
64. Taylor, G. I., The dispersion of matter in turbulent flow through a pipe, *Proc. R. Soc. London. Ser. A,* 223, 446, 1954.
65. Emerson, J. H., Apparatus for Vibrating Portions of a Patients Airway; U.S. Patent Number 2918917; Dec. 29, 1959.
66. Bohn, D. J., Miyasaka, K., Marchak, B. E., et al., Ventilation by high-frequency oscillation, *J. Appl. Physiol.,* 48, 710, 1980.
67. Butler, W. J., Bohn, D. J., Bryan, A. C., et al., Ventilation by high-frequency oscillation in humans, *Anesth. Analg.,* 59, 577, 1980.
68. Slutsky, A. S., Drazen, J. M., Ingram, R. H., et al., Effective pulmonary ventilation with small-volume oscillations at high frequency, *Science,* 209, 609, 1980.
69. Slutsky, A. S., Kamm, R. D., Rossing, T. H., et al., Effects of frequency, tidal volume, and lung volume on CO_2 elimination in dogs by high frequency (2—30 Hz), low tidal volume ventilation, *J. Clin. Invest.,* 68, 1475, 1981.
70. Ngeow, Y. K. and Mitzner, W., A new system for ventilating with high-frequency oscillation, *J. Appl. Physiol.,* 53, 1638, 1982.

71. Boynton, B. R., Mannino, F. L., Davis, R. F., et al., Combined high-frequency oscillatory ventilation and intermittent mandatory ventilation in critically Ill neonates, *J. Pediatr.*, 105, 297, 1984.
72. Rossing, T. H., Solway, J., Saari, A. F., et al., Influence of the endotracheal tube on CO_2 transport during high frequency ventilation, *Am. Rev. Respir. Dis.*, 129, 54, 1984.
73. Fletcher, P. R. and Epstein, R. A., Measurement of alveolar pressures during HFV, *Anesthesiology*, 55, A358, 1981.
74. Fletcher, P. R., Alveolar pressures during high frequency ventilation, in *Perspectives in High Frequency Ventilation*, Scheck, P. A., Sjstrand, U. H., and Smith, R. B., Eds., Martinus Nijhoff, Boston, 1983.
75. Rossing, T. H., Slutsky, A. S., Lehr, J. L., et al., Tidal volume and frequency dependence of carbon dioxide elimination by high-frequency ventilation, *N. Engl. J. Med.*, 305, 1375, 1981.
76. Kolton, M., Cattran, C., Bryan, A. C., et al., High frequency oscillation and mean lung volume, *Anesthesiology*, 55, A353, 1981.
77. Suwa, K. and Tagami, M., Ventilatory volume and pressure required for oscillatory ventilation in dogs, *Jap. J. Physiol.*, 32, 443, 1982.
78. Helperin, S. W. and Waskow, W. H., Emerson wrap-around chest respirator for use in bronchoscopy and laryngoscopy, *Anesth. Analg.*, 38, 444, 1959.
79. Green, R. A. and Coleman, D. J., Cuirass respirator for endoscopy, *Anaesthesia*, 10, 369, 1955.
80. Johnson, D. L., Various aspects of infrasound, *Proc. Colloque Int. sur les Infra-Sons*, September, 24—27, CNET, Moulineaux, France, 1973, 337.
81. Ward, H. E., Power, J. H. T., and Nicholas, T. E., High-frequency oscillations via the pleural surface: an alterative mode of ventilation?, *J. Appl. Physiol.*, 54, 427, 1983.
82. Bitterman, H., Kerem, D., Shabtai, Y., et al., Respiration maintained by externally applied vibration and tracheal insufflation in the cat, *Anesth. Analg.*, 62, 33, 1983.
83. Zidulka, A., Gross, D., Minami, H., et al., Ventilation by high-frequency chest wall compression in dogs with normal lungs, *Am. Rev. Respir. Dis.*, 127, 709, 1983.
84. Medical Device Amendments of 1976: Public Law 94-295, May 28, 1976.
85. Everything You Always Wanted to Know About the Medical Device Ammendments . . . and Weren't Afraid to Ask, HEW Publication No. (FDA) 77-5006, U.S. Department of Health, Education, and Welfare; Public Health Service; Food and Drug Administration; Bureau of Medical Devices; Silver Spring, Md., 1977.
86. Gluck, M. S., The regulation of medical devices by the FDA, *J. Clin. Monitoring*, in press.

Chapter 9

SELECTION OF MECHANICAL VENTILATORY SUPPORT BASED ON RESPIRATORY PATHOPHYSIOLOGY*

Graziano C. Carlon and Arthur H. Combs

Mechanical ventilation has represented the cornerstone of therapy of respiratory insufficiency and respiratory failure for the last three decades. The evolution of mechanical ventilation began with attempts to duplicate natural processes. This approach may not have been the most efficient, but it did have innumerable historical precedents. In the early development of the airplane, many designs attempted unsuccessfully to achieve flight by reproducing the beat of the wings of birds. The first cars were merely horsedrawn carriages to which a combustion engine had been added. Even with the most daring of innovations, there seemed to be a tendency to incorporate as many pre-existing solutions as possible. The development of mechanical ventilators did not escape this general tendency, as initial designs attempted to reproduce the principles of spontaneous breathing. The lungs, located in the sealed thoracic cavity, are covered by the visceral pleura. The visceral pleura is intimately associated with the thoracic parietal pleura through a thin layer of fluid which provides a very high surface tension. Thus, any change of shape involving the chest wall or diaphragm necessarily affects the lungs.

During inspiration, the thoracic cavity and the lungs increase in volume, acting as bellows and decreasing pressure in the intrapleural space and alveoli. Gases then flow from the environment at atmospheric pressure to the alveoli. The first mechanical ventilators for long term support were designed to expand the chest wall.[1] Patients were inserted into a container which could be tightly sealed to permit generation of negative pressure. Each cycle of the ventilator passively expanded the chest wall, and therefore, the lungs. Although this method closely reproduced spontaneous breathing, its limitations were very substantial. Even disregarding the clumsiness of the apparatus and the difficulty of rendering proper nursing care, the degree of negative pressure which could be generated was insufficient to expand markedly uncompliant lungs in severe forms of acute respiratory failure. Nonetheless, the iron lung was very useful for patients with neuromuscular deficits,[2] and has still been used recently both in children[3] and adults[4] with *Pneumocystis carinii* pneumonia.

The next step in the evolution of mechanical ventilators was the development of instruments which expanded the lungs by increasing alveolar pressure, rather than by decreasing intrapleural pressure. Although modern volume-cycled ventilators are substantially more efficient, flexible, and safer than those introduced in the 1950s,[5,6] the basic principles of operation have not changed. The major conceptual changes include the application of PEEP[7-9] and IMV.[10-14]

PEEP should be hailed as the first attempt to manage acute respiratory failure on the basis of its pathophysiology.[15-20] The reader is also referred to many comprehensive reviews over the past 10 years.[21-35] In respiratory failure, the major source of hypoxemia is the presence of severe ventilation/perfusion inequality.[25,26] This is caused by functional or anatomical collapse of alveoli and terminal respiratory units, precluding gas exchange within areas of the lungs which are still perfused. The measurable results of these changes are a progressive increase in the closing volume and a simultaneous

* The authors gratefully acknowledge Ms. Clara Ducham for expert editorial assistance in the preparation of this manuscript.

decrease in FRC. While perfusion is maintained, the areas of functional collapse contribute to increasing shunt fraction ($\dot{Q}s/\dot{Q}t$) and thus to hypoxemia. The conceptual basis of PEEP is marvelously efficient in its simplicity: by raising the pressure within the airways and the aveoli to a value approximating critical closing pressure, alveolar collapse at the end of each expiration should be prevented, maintaining adequate gas exchange throughout the entire respiratory cycle. From this consideration derives an immediate major difference between intermittent positive pressure ventilation (IPPV) and IPPV with PEEP. In the former (IPPV alone), alveoli may be opened by high peak inspiratory pressures, but they will be allowed to collapse again during exhalation as airway pressure falls to atmospheric. Characteristically, the inspiratory phase represents less than one half (and frequently one third or less) of each respiratory cycle. Even those alveoli successfully recruited by an IPPV breath will be available for gas exchange only a fraction of each breath, while contributing to venous admixture during the remaining time. IPPV with PEEP not only increases the number of alveoli that at any one time are available for gas exchange, but more significantly, substantially expands the time during which alveoli functionally exchange gases. In essence, PEEP changes the time constant of alveolar units, increasing speed and efficiency of gas exchange.

It is still surprising to consider the degree of opposition which the application of PEEP encountered for many years.[40,44] Many respected authors with credentials in the management of respiratory failure had no hesitation in placing categorical and arbitrary upper limits to the maximum level of PEEP[41-43] that could be safely administered. This approach not only contradicts the principle that physiologic functions are not amenable to rigorous limitations, but also fails to recognize that it is inherent to the concept of PEEP therapy that levels administered should be proportional to the severity of the lung injury.[36]

At the other extreme, some authors have proposed the application of very high levels of PEEP where necessary, as high as 40 to 60 cm H_2O.[36-38] This approach did not encounter much favor, since very few patients could objectively benefit from it. A major limitation to the application of high PEEP is that even patients with very severe forms of respiratory failure may have different degrees of involvement of different areas of the lung. Application of a uniform mode of therapy may result in as much injury to the sections of the lung which do not need it as benefits to those which do.[34] Complex techniques, such as separate lung ventilation,[45,46] have been proposed in some instances of differential lung injury, but they too are of objective benefit for only a limited number of patients.[47]

Despite an increased understanding of the pathophysiology of respiratory failure[19,21,23,30,32,48-56] and technical advances in the design of mechanical ventilators, the mortality rate associated with the disease is still high.[57,58] Although statistics vary substantially, since different authors use different criteria to define respiratory failure,[23,33,149] 30 to 60% of patients die when severe hypoxemia requiring mechanical respiratory support develops.

Most patients improve, at least temporarily, when mechanical ventilation is instituted; but in some patients therapeutic interventions aimed at increasing FRC may be accompanied by deterioration of blood gases.[39] In rare cases, failure may be readily explained by substantial differences in the degree of involvement of the lungs[39,45-47] or by the presence of major airway disruption.[59] In most cases, however, obvious reasons are not apparent.[60,61] Increasing convective gas flow, using large volumes and pressures, may not be sufficient when maldistribution of ventilation and perfusion are at the basis of respiratory failure. In other words, if spontaneous ventilation does not deliver gases to areas of the lungs which need to be ventilated, a mechanical device operating on the same general principles of convection may also fail. Although intriguing, this theory has never been satisfactorily proven, since the necessary measurements — lung volume and regional ventilation/perfusion ratio — cannot be easily obtained. In some disease entities, the inadequacies of conventional mechanical support have a better pathophysiologic justification. In bullous emphysema, for example, total lung compliance may be increased, even though areas affected by a pneumonic process may have a lower compliance. In these patients, mechanical methods of ventilation which uniformly increase airway pressure will over-distend the bullous areas while underventilating the injured, uncompliant portions of the lungs. Bullous areas already have a very high $\dot{V}/\dot{Q}$ which will be further augmented by positive pressure ventilation. Accordingly, much of any given tidal breath will be wasted as the compliant bullae act as anatomical dead space, increasing the ratio of dead space to tidal volume (V_D/V_T). Areas of the lung with intact perfusion may be denied ventilation because their compliance is low by comparison. This disease has the same pathophysiologic problems as unilateral lung injury. Correction by the use of two ventilators is, however, impossible, since bullae usually affect both lungs. Interstitial lung disease associated with collagen deposition is becoming more common with the increased use of radiotherapy and pulmonary-toxic chemotherapy.[61] This process may also prevent the successful use of positive pressure ventilation. Alveoli encased by fibrotic tissue cannot be expanded. By instituting positive pressure ventilation, lung disruption, rather than increasing, FRC, may be the consequence of high peak inspiratory pressures.

Finally, it is accepted by most authors that elevated peak inspiratory pressures will increase extravascular lung water[41,62-65] and damge surfactant function,[66] again justifying some of the concern about conventional mechanical ventilation.

The high mortality associated with acute respiratory failure has spurred the research of alternative modalities to be used when conventional mechanical ventilation fails. In past years great hopes had been placed on extracorporeal membrane oxygenation support (ECMO),[67] a technique to bypass the lungs and provide gas exchange outside the body. The results of the ECMO cooperative study were highly unsatisfactory,[68,69] with a mortality rate exceeding 90% in those patients sufficiently ill to justify utilization of the extremely expensive technique.

More recently, a different approach has been proposed, with the use of mechanical ventilators operating on principles somewhat different from those of conventional devices. HFV employs high breathing frequencies and reduced tidal volumes which are at times less than anatomical dead space. The concept that gas exchange can be maintained at breathing rates far higher than the physiologic range of 10 to 30 breaths/min is not new. Some such experiments were reported as early as 1915.[70] However, clinical investigations on the applicability of HFV in respiratory failure date only to 1977.[71] A ventilator was designed in 1967, with the specific purpose of minimizing interference with cardiac function.[72,73] The authors broke new ground with their decision to design the ventilator based on a specific function of performance rather than accepting the notion that a mechanism delivered very small tidal volumes, at rates of 60 to 100 breaths/min; the method was called HFPPV. This ventilator is now well known, and its merits and disadvantages have been extensively investigated.[74-84] A thorough discussion of HFPPV would not be appropriate here, but the interested reader may refer to many authoritative reviews.[85-92] It must be emphasized that more than the ventilator itself, the concept that a mechanical system need not reproduce natural physiologic mechanism to obtain comparable results, is the most valuable result of this research.

HFJV, although first described many years ago,[93,94] has only become popular in the last 6 to 7 years The first paper of substantial clinical interest described the utilization of HFJV to provide mechanical respiration to dogs without the need of an endotracheal tube.[95,96] Studies on HFJV have been directed toward three major areas: definition of the ideal technical characteristics for a jet ventilator, interactions between the ventilator and the patient, and identification of patients most likely to benefit from HFJV.

Ideally, mechanical ventilation should maintain arterial oxygenation and CO_2 clearance, while interfering minimally with the function of other organs and systems. This holds equally true for conventional and high frequency ventilators. When evaluating HFJV, each component which may affect delivery to the patient must be considered separately. These components include the pressure source, the gating mechanism, the inspiratory line, and the injector cannula.

The pressure source delivers gases to the gating mechanism. Under normal circumstances, the pressure source is the centralized oxygen and air supplies of the hospital, but any system which provides compressed gases will suffice. The minimum pressure required varies with the type of ventilator. Pneumatic and fluidic jet ventilators[97-99] which utilize gas pressure to direct gas flow and control ventilator function generally require higher operating pressure than electronic[100,113] or mechanical jet ventilators. When the gas source delivers a mixture of air and oxygen, as is most commonly the case, pressure variations must be controlled to avoid substantial inaccuracies in the concentration of oxygen (FiO_2). Some air-oxygen blenders have an unpredictable output when gas pressure varies. It is desirable to frequently test the accuracy of the oxygen concentration delivered, using a polarographic oxygen analyzer or other similarly accurate method.[112] In most papers published in the U.S.; the pressure with which the gases are delivered is expressed in pounds per square inch (psi). The conversion factor is 1 psi = 70.4 cm H_2O = 51.7 mmHg. All studies reported thus far indicate that very rarely is a gas pressure exceeding 50 psi necessary to maintain adequate ventilation.[103,104] This value is within the range of the centralized oxygen supply system of most hospitals and most regulators on compressed medical gas cylinders.

Gases delivered from the central source under pressure must be gated before reaching the patient. Gating is the fundamental function of a jet ventilator. Whether this operation is performed by a mechanical or pneumatic system, the gating mechanism determines the number of cycles (respiratory rate, breaths/min) and, within each cycle, the percentage of time during which gas flow to the patient is allowed ("on time"), the latter being referred to as the duty cycle. For instance, if respiratory rate is 100 breaths/min and inspiratory time is 33%, during each cycle the gate is open for 200 msec and closed for 400 msec (60 sec/100 BPM = 600 msec/c). It can be immediately derived from these considerations that fast and accurate function of the gating mechanism is fundamental in determining the efficiency of gas delivery. Even at the relatively low rate of 100 breaths/min, a gate mechanism requiring 20 msec to open or close would add a significant error factor to the determination of inspiratory/expiratory time (20 msec/c × 100 c = 2 sec/min used solely to operate gate). Utilizing a 33% inspiratory time means that only 20 sec of each minute the ventilator is delivering gases to the patient. An error of 2 sec, wasted on gate operation, would represent a 10% reduction in minute ventilation.[100] Furthermore, whenever the valve is partially open or partially closed, gas pressure in the inspiratory line is affected, influencing gas flow through the injector cannula, and thus the ratio of directly delivered gases to entrainment.[104] In the design of a jet ventilator, a nearly instantaneous gating mechanism should always be used, in order to provide an almost perfectly square inspiratory waveform.[100-103,105] (Figures 1 and 2.)

The inspiratory line is composed of the tubing between the gating mechanism and the injector cannula. This component of a jet ventilator must also conform to strict criteria, to provide reliable gas delivery. As previously indicated, operational pressures are orders of magnitude higher than those normally present in the inspiratory line of a conventional ventilator, at times, more than three atmospheres. Even a relatively low

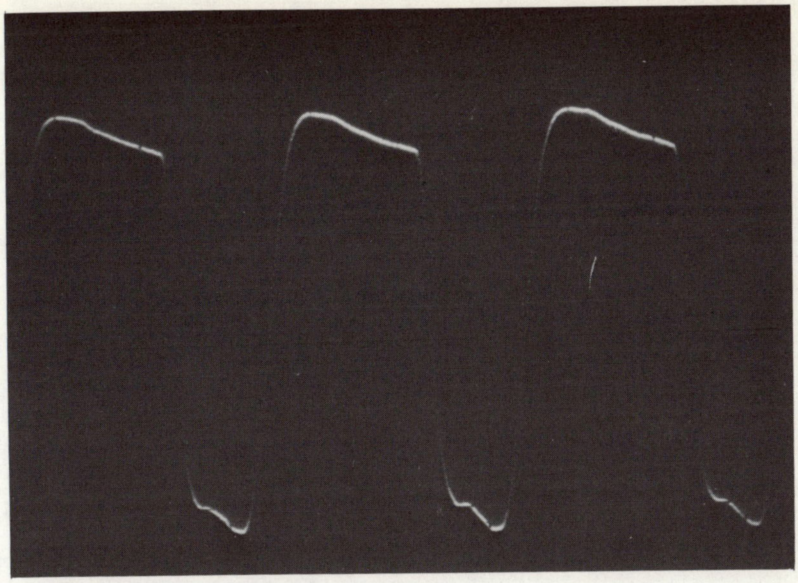

Driving Pressure:	40	psig
Cannula Diameter:	1.62	mm
Resistance:	5	cm H_2O/L/sec
Compliance:	50	ml/cm H_2O
PEEP:	$\overline{0}$	cm H_2O
Entertainment:	Demand Valve	
V_t:	280	ml
PaW:	50	cm H_2O
Resp. Rate:	100	breaths/min

FIGURE 1. At a frequency of 100 breaths/min and an inspiratory/expiratory ratio of 1:2, each solenoid valve duty cycle lasts approximately 200 msec. The airway pressure measured at the cannula tip demonstrates an almost instantaneous rise and a plateau lasting for most of the inspiration.

driving pressure, such as 15 psi, which can effectively support a patient with normal lungs, is equivalent to 1000 cm H_2O, or 30 times higher than pressures in the inspiratory line of a conventional ventilator. At such pressures, the compressible volume of the gases in the tubing becomes very significant. In conventional ventilators, compressible volumes of 1.5 to 3.5 mℓ/cm H_2O are considered normal. This figure takes into account both the effect of Boyle's law on the volume of gases present in the inspiratory line and the deformatory of the tubing itself. On HFV, these values would result in very large gas loss to volume compression, essentially negating gas delivery to the patient. Even a very small compressible volume, such as 0.1 mℓ/cm H_2O, would still account for a tidal volume loss up to 100 mℓ at a driving pressure of 15 psi (1000 cm H_2O 0.1 mℓ/cm H_2O = 100 mℓ lost). Even more significant than the actual reduction in tidal volume is the change of pressure waveform associated with compliant

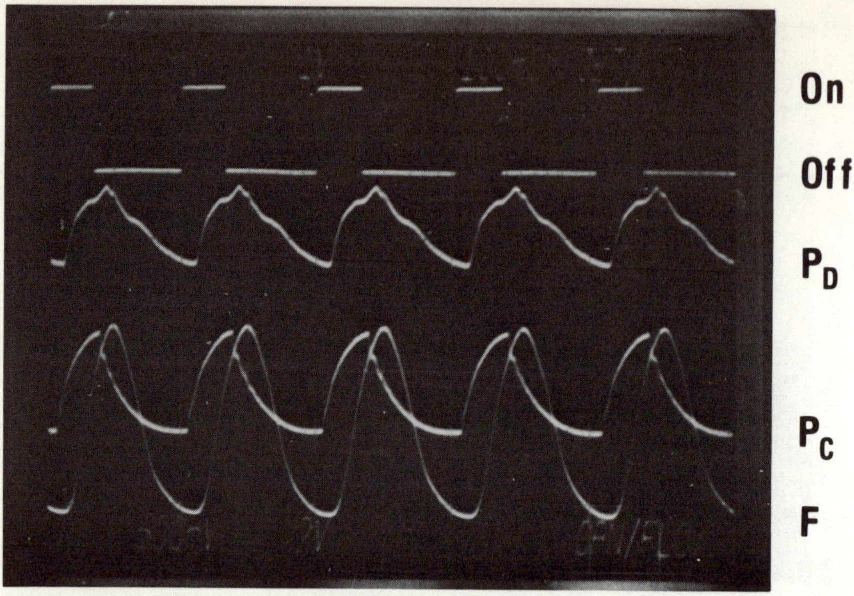

Rate(P)	**300 breaths/min**
P_D	**Driving Pressure**
P_C	**Pressure-Cannula Tip**
F	**Flow**
On	**Jet Solenoid Duty Cycle On**
Off	**Jet Solenoid Duty Cycle Off**

FIGURE 2. At 300 breaths/min, there is a delay between the opening of the injector cannula and the detection of peak inspiratory pressure in the inspiratory line and at the cannula tip. Gas flows reported here are simply the electrical output from a Hans-Rudolph pneumotachograph and do not represent measurable tidal volume.

tubing.[103] Initial pressure rise, after the opening of the solenoid valve is slowed because part of the energy is dissipated to compress gases already present in the inspiratory line. When the solenoid valve closes, the compressed gases remaining in the inspiratory line will maintain a residual pressure at the injector cannula and will therefore prolong gas flow through the injector cannula. As a result, the pressure waveform is modified from square to sinusoidal.[100-102,105] (Figure 3.) This in turn will reduce the magnitude of entrainment, which is dependent on gas flow velocity and pressure gradient at the cannula nozzle,[107,108] and may also contribute to an unplanned level of PEEP.[96,103,106,118]

To prevent or at least minimize these problems, three design characteristics of the inspiratory line are desirable, all of which contribute to a reduction in the compressible volume. First, the tubing should be as short as is practical. Second, it should be made of a virtually undeformable material such as Teflon (0.005 mℓ/cm H_2O). Lastly, the diameter of the tubing should be only three to four times that of the injector cannula (0.6 cm = 4 × 0.162; see below). Since resistances are proportional to the fourth power of the radius when flow is laminar, (Poiseuille's Law: resistance = (8 × tube length × gas viscosity)/(Pi × tube radius^4))[109] and since the tubing and injector are in series, this

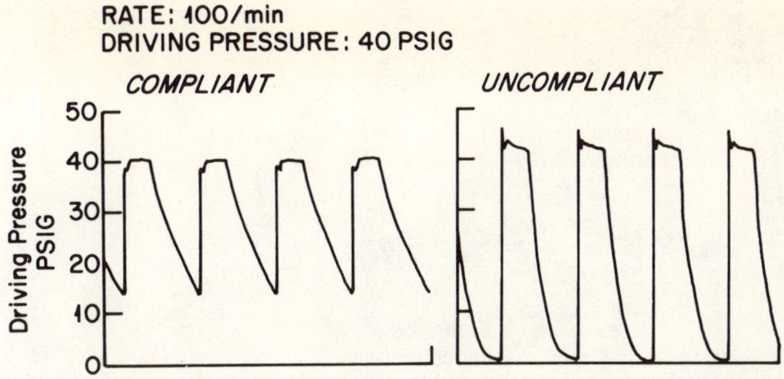

FIGURE 3. Effect of a compliant or uncompliant inspiratory line on inspiratory pressure waveform motion. Notice the residual end-expiratory pressure, between solenoid valve duty cycles, with the compliant tubings.

restricts all meaningful resistance of the system to the injector cannula. Short length, small radius tubing should minimize compressible volume.

The solenoid valve has a central and critical role in the function of the jet ventilator. It is responsible for control of the respirator frequency as well as the duty cycle (inspiratory/expiratory ratio). At a frequency of 100 bpm, the solenoid will open and close 144,000 times per day. Absolute reliability over many millions of cycles is an essential characteristic of any gating mechanism. Fortunately, solenoid valves certified for as many as 100 million cycles are commercially available.[100]

The injector cannula also plays a critical role as it determines gas pressure and velocity. These in turn, are major determinants of gas entrainment. It follows then, that the injector cannula has a major influence on tidal volume delivered under a given set of conditions. A number of investigators have attempted to define the characteristics of an ideal injector cannula.[100-106,110,111,113-116] Factors which have been considered include: the diameter and length of the cannula, the ratio between the cross-sectional surface of the cannula and that of the tube that contains it (cannula:exhaust lumen ratio), the axial orientation of the cannula within the tube, the distance between the injector cannula tip and the entrainment source (if any), and the distance of the injector cannula tip from the carina.

Available bench tests, animal experiments and human studies permit a number of conclusions. The range of diameters of injectors cannulas in use is 1 to 2 mm, with a strong indication that cannulas with a diameter less than 1.5 mm may not provide adequate gas flow for patients with severe respiratory failure.[102,104,106] The length of the injector cannula does not seem to be of major signifcance, except when the distance between the tip of the cannula and the entrainment source affects gas entrainment. When a critical distance between injector cannula tip and additional gas source is exceeded, minimal increments drastically reduce entrainment.[101,115] (Figure 4.) Entrainment is also frequently absent when gas delivery takes place through the extruded lumen of an endotracheal tube, with the opening a few centimeters from its distal end.[105,114] Ideal ratios between the injector cannula lumen and endotracheal tube cross-sectional areas have been established — entrainment and CO_2 clearance are significantly impaired when this ratio falls below 1:6.[104,105,119] The explanation proposed is that a large injector cannula placed inside a small endotracheal tube is a source of considerable local turbulence, reducing foward gas motion and increasing rebreathing. A measurable difference in entrainment, although of questionable clincal significance, can be observed even with large endotracheal tubes. For example, reducing the tube

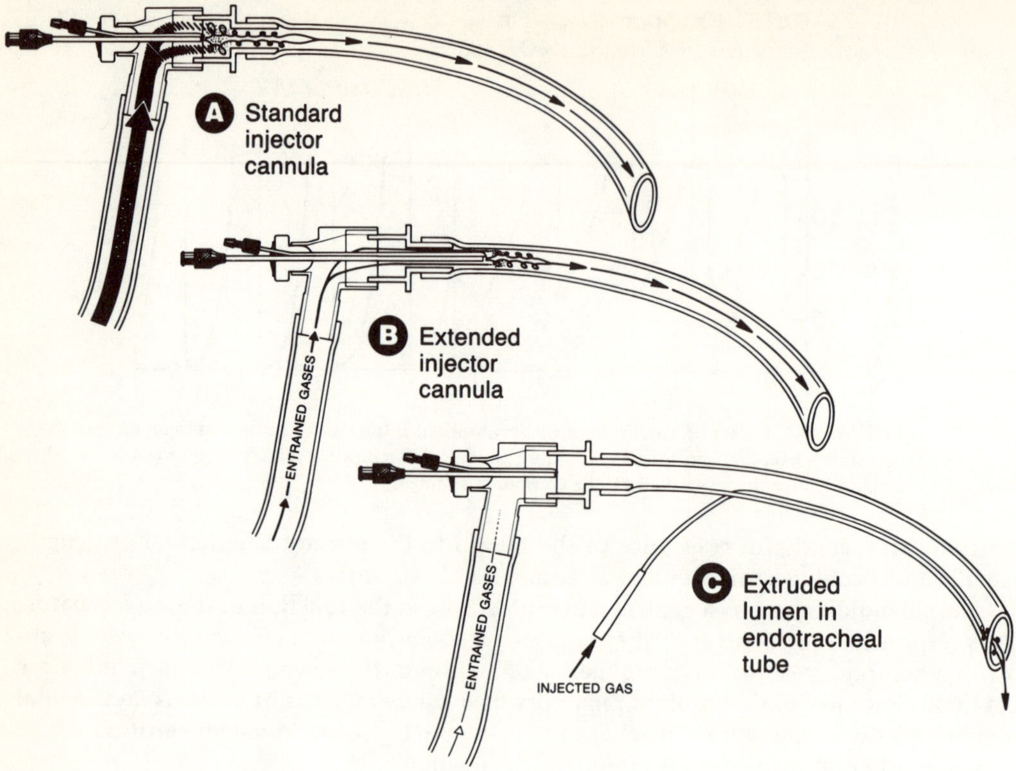

FIGURE 4. Schematic representation of the varying relationship between injector cannula and entrained volume, based on spatial location of the entrainment port.

diameter from 10 to 7 mm results in decreased gas entrainment by 15 to 20%,[101] even though the ratios of injector cannula-to-endotracheal tube cross-sectional area are 40:1 and 20:1. (Figures 5 and 6.) In summary, it appears that the most effective placement of the injector cannulas is central axial, inserted at the proximal end of the endotracheal tube and with the tip in close proximity to the source of entrainment.

The actual role played by entrainment in maintaining adequate gas exchange during HFJV, and therefore its clinical relevance, has not been determined. Bench tests suggest that the application of even relatively small loads downstream, represented by either increased resistance or decreased compliance distal to the injector cannula, drastically reduces entrainment.[101,102,111,116,120] A sharp increase in resistance virtually eliminates entrainment.[101]

The consequences of these observations on clinical applications of HFJV are substantial. Disease characterized by a drastic reduction of the distal airway load will greatly benefit by administration of HFJV with unrestricted entrainment. One such condition is a major airway disruption, as in bronchopleural or tracheoesophageal fistula. The airway leak represents an alternative path with very high compliance for each tidal volume, placed in parallel with the alveoli. On HFJV, the higher compliance and the reduction of downstream impedance associated with higher cycle frequencies will increase entrainment. Volume losses through the pathologic opening will be compensated for by enhanced entrainment without encroaching on the minute ventilation of the lungs. The power peak airway pressures prevent physical enlargement of the pathologic opening, further increasing the effectiveness of HFJV in such conditions. Electrical circuit analogs[101,102,121,147] of the physical model of airway disruption have been proposed, providing theoretical support for clinical observations.[122-133,148] Ade-

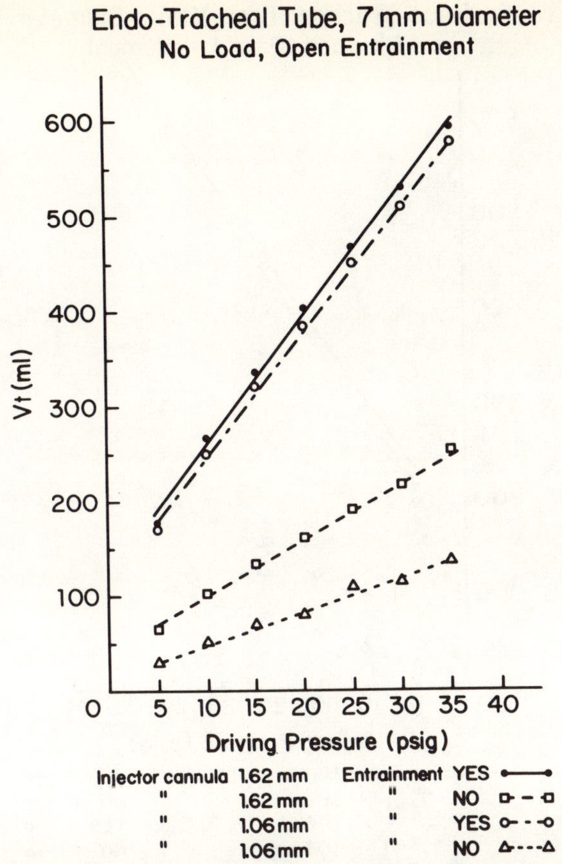

FIGURE 5. Tidal volume, measured in the presence or absence of entrainment, with injector cannulas of two different diameters and an endotracheal tube of either 7 or 10 cm diameter. The reduction of entrainment at constant tidal volume delivered through the injector cannula, is evident with the smaller endotracheal tube.

quate gas exchange can be maintained on HFJV even in the presence of airway leaks as large as the cross-sectional area of the trachea itself.[126,133]

In patients with acute respiratory failure, depending on the etiology, entrainment is often less important. Even with airway resistances within normal range (5 cm H_2O/L/sec) and a modest reduction of compliance (50 mℓ/cm H_2O), as are observed in the mildest forms of acute respiratory failure, entrainment does not represent more than 25 to 30% of total delivered volume.[101,111,116] (Figure 7.) With larger increases in airway resistance or reductions in compliance, as are seen in the more severe forms of respiratory failure, entrainment is practically abolished.[101,104,106,110,111] (Figure 8.)

Entrainment is an extremely labile variable, being affected by all control variables — frequency driving pressure, duty cycle and cannula size — as well as by physiological variables — notably resistance and compliance. Under conditions in which entrainment contributes little to minute ventilation, tidal volume can be determined more precisely as it largely represents gas flow through the injector cannula itself. Since the injector represents the most significant resistance in the entire ventilator-patient system, no change in the condition of the lungs could significantly affect tidal volume. The absence of entrainment, however, is associated with increased airway pressure at a given

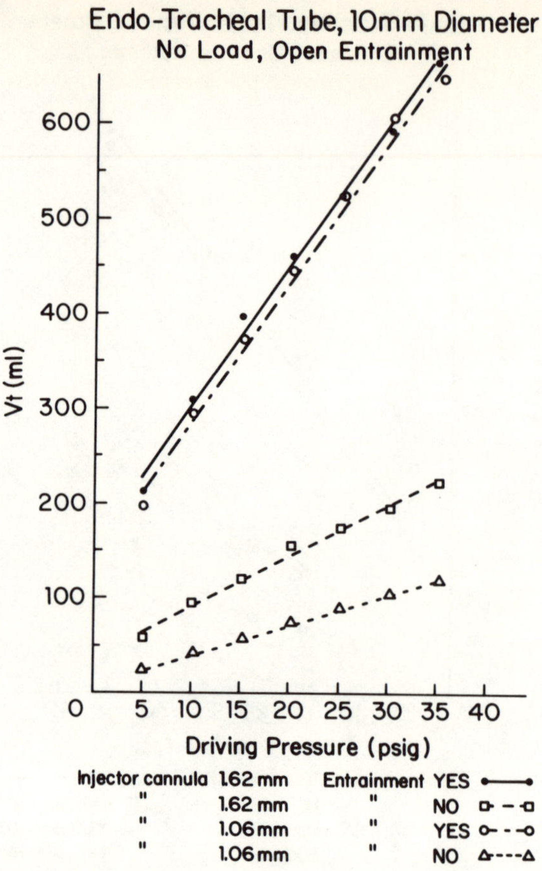

FIGURE 6. Tidal volume, measured in the presence or absence of entrainment, with injector cannulas of two different diameters and an endotracheal tube of either 7 or 10 cm diameter. The reduction of entrainment, at constant tidal volume delivered through the injector cannula, is evident with the smaller endotracheal tube.

level of ventilation.[101] This is because the moderating affect of momentum and kinetic energy transfer between injector and entrained gases is a function of their velocity ($KE = 1/2\ mv^2$) which is, in turn, inversely proportional to cannula size (i.e., the smaller the cannula, the higher the velocity at any given driving pressure). This accounts in large measure for the greater entrainment seen with smaller injector cannulas. In systems where entrainment was unimpeded, tidal volumes increased only twofold with an increase in cannula size from 1.02 to 1.62 mm, despite a sixfold decrease in resistance.[101-104,106,110]

An integrated depiction of HFJV combines the effects of physiological variables and the law of conservation of energy and momentum. Gases flowing from the injector have a certain momentum and kinetic energy based on their mass and velocity. When these rapidly flowing gases impact on the immobile gases present in the endotracheal tube (or proximal airways), a forward motion in the direction of the net vector of gas flow is generated, thus initiating convective gas flow. (Figure 9.) The larger the volume of gases in the upper airway compared to the volume of flow through the injector cannula, the more rapidly the pressure and velocity of the two gas masses will equalize. At the same time, a progressively larger volume of gases moves down the airways at

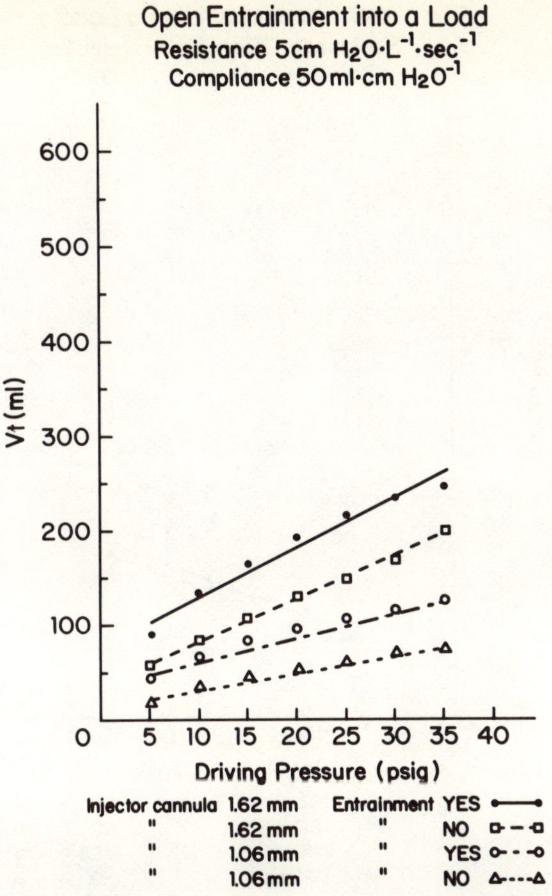

FIGURE 7. A minimal increase of resistance and compliance sharply reduces entrained volume and, to a much less degree, gas flow directly delivered through the injector cannula.

decreasing speed and pressure, turbulence decreases and the velocity profile assumes the shape of a cone characteristic of laminar flow.[134] Entrainment decreases flow rate, since the larger the total volume (mass) of gases moved, the lower the ultimate velocity ($KE = 1/2\ mv^2$). Accordingly, the duration of inspiration is substantially larger in the lower airways than through the injector cannula. The basic physiological principle that pressure is directly related to flow rate is respected. Moreover, the cone-shaped flow velocity profile acquired by inspiratory gases within the airways also provides a rational explanation for the adequacy of gas exchange obtained despite small tidal volumes — volumes which would normally be insufficient with conventional methods of support.[135-137] These considerations help to explain the lower airway pressure observed.

Clinical studies indicate that tidal volumes of 3 to 4.5 mℓ/kg, approximately one third of those required with conventional ventilators, maintain eucapnia even in the presence of severe respiratory failure.[60,101,014,106,138,139] The cone-shaped flow velocity profile allows a portion of a given tidal volume to move distally down the airways with each subsequent breath (inspiration) (Figure 10.) Since the exhalation velocity profile is also cone-shaped,[136] a transitional volume of fresh gases which were delivered but not exhaled will remain within the airways after each tidal exchange. With each ensuing breath, these gases will be moved further down the airway. It will then be only a matter

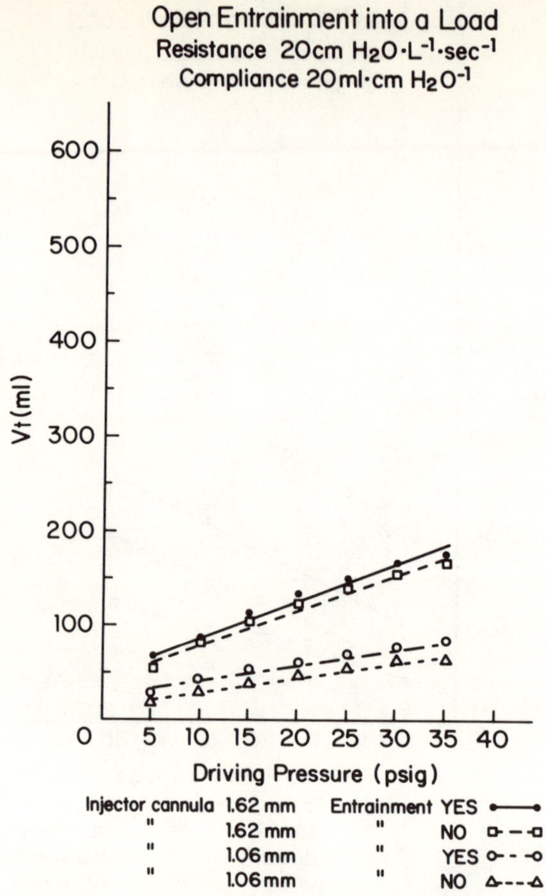

FIGURE 8. A further sharp increase in resistance and decrease in compliance effectively eliminates entrainment, although gas volume delivered through the injector cannula is essentially unchanged.

of time until a steady state, with continuous availability of fresh gases at the alveolar level is achieved. The key to understanding the process of gas exchange is to appreciate that fresh alveolar gases need not necessarily derive from the tidal volume of the last breath delivered, but may be composed of gases inhaled over a number of breaths. This mechanism, for which there is solid mathematical support,[142] indicates that convective mechanisms can explain gas exchange at the alveolar level on HFJV,[140] without the need to postulate enhanced diffusion,[141,143] — a mechanism which may be inadequate at the frequencies applicable to HFJV.

In the standard physical model of a jet injector the volume of space which jet flow enters after leaving the injector cannula is called the mixing chamber. In clinical settings, this is usually the endotrachela tube. Local conditions of the mixing chamber, as well as changes in control variables, will greatly affect the characterstics of the jet flow. It is here that the influences of cycle frequency and duty cycle determine the physicologic consequences and clinical efficacy of HFJV.[105,144]

From the description of the jet ventilator, it can be derived that an increase in respiratory rate, unlike conventional volume-cycled ventilation, does not necessarily imply an increase in minute volume.[140] The opposite may at times be true. Minute volume depends most directly on the length of time the solenoid valve remains open, and on

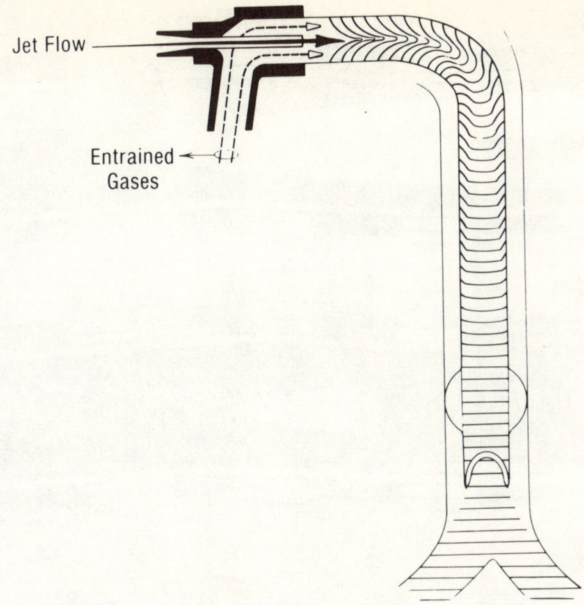

FIGURE 9. Graphic representation of the physics of jet mixing and entrainment. A progressively larger volume of gases moves down the airway with progressively decreasing speed and pressure.

entrainment. When entrainment is not permitted, tidal volume is linearly related to inspiratory time, minute ventilation increasing with inspiratory/expiratory ratio, rather than with tidal volume per se. All studies thus far performed confirm that the relationship between inspiratory/expiratory (I:E) ratio and tidal volume is different when entrainment is allowed.[100,101,104,105,111,144]

Entrainment depends on gas velocity and pressure at the jet nozzle, with velocity playing the most important role. The differences between the velocity and pressure of gases exiting from the injector cannula and the gases already present in the upper airways steadily decrease after flow is initiated, as a consequence of the transfer of momentum and kinetic energy from jet flow to the immobile gases in the upper airways. Increasing I:E ratio, therefore, will not result in a linear increase of tidal volume. When pressure in the upper airways increases, entrainment will proportionally decrease.[101,104] Prolongation of I:E ratio can result in higher inspiratory pressure because mean flow rate is higher, thus decreasing entrainment and therefore, tidal volume. Prolongation of inspiration necessarily decreases expiratory time and as a consequence may produce distal alveolar gas trapping.[101,118,144,145] This phenomenon can also increase airway pressure and, thus, significantly limit entrainment and tidal volume.

For reasons relating largely to the physical limitations of the gating mechanism, jet ventilators do not effectively operate at frequencies exceeding 300 breaths/min.[100,101,106] Most investigators utilize frequencies between 100 and 500 breaths/min.[124,125,139] It is consistently observed that, at higher rates, CO_2 clearance deteriorates,[138,140,144,146] even when minute ventilation increases, and mean airway and end-expiratory airway pressures increase.[104,118,145] High respiratory rates are associated with increased turbulence in the proximal airways and more air trapping in the distal airways, resulting in poor alveolar gas exchange and increased mean transpulmonary pressure, respectively. In theory, gas trapping may increase functional residual capacity and therefore improve oxygenation,[145] but this beneficial effect may be overshadowed by negative effects on CO_2 elimination and cardiac function.

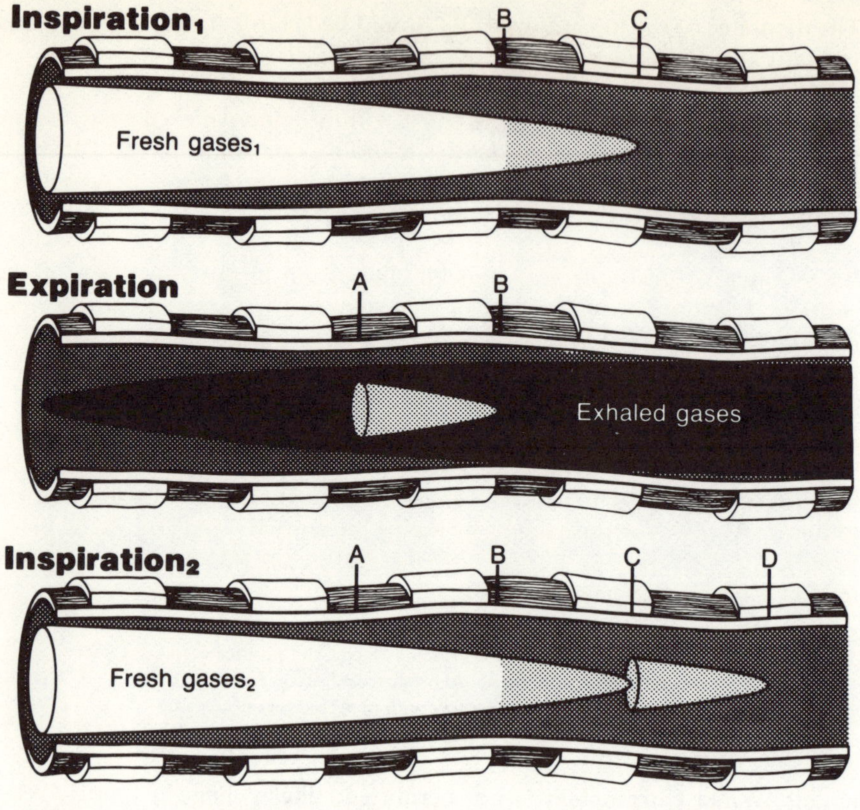

FIGURE 10. Schematic representation suggesting how alveolar gas exchange on HFV may be explained on the basis of conventional convective mechanisms, as proposed by Jaeger. After each breath a residual volume of fresh gases remains in the airways and is moved distally by the next breath. After a finite number of breaths, a steady state will be reached, where fresh gas continuously reaches the alveolar level.

It is readily apparent that clinical effectiveness of HFJV will be directly dependent on the physiologic consequences of how it is applied. The mechanical components themselves, the design variables, and the manipulation of control variables must be integrated and tailored to the clinical setting. Based on theoretical, experimental and available clinical information, we may formulate a number of recommendations.[101,145]

- HFJV should be connected to an adjustable pressure source, which can operate at 50 psi or higher.
- The gating mechanism should have an almost instantaneous response, enabling the ventilator to function efficiently at frequencies as high as 300 breaths/min.
- The inspiratory line should have its internal compressible volume reduced as much as possible, and should be made of virtually noncompliant material.
- The injector cannula should be inserted at the proximal end of the endotracheal tube, be oriented coaxially and in its exact center.
- The ratio between the injector cannula and endotracheal tube cross-sectional areas (injector:exhaust area) should minimize gas trapping, and should never be less than 1:6.

- The diameter of the injector cannula should be 1.5 to 2.0 mm, and should provide virtually the entire resistance of the inspiratory circuit.

- Respiratory rate should be maintained within limits which do not substantially increase airway pressure and/or gas trapping (generally $\leq$ 150 BPM). Similar considerations apply to the adjustment of the duty cycle (I:E ratio). I:E ratio should never exceed 1:1.

- Entrainment is desirable and clinically important in the presence of airway disruption. It often does not, nor can it be expected to, play an equally significant role in the presence of severe respiratory failure. Adjustments of minute ventilation must take these differences among clinical settings into account.

- The role of HFJV in the management of patients with various forms of respiratory insufficiency and respiratory failure has not yet been fully elucidated. A better understanding of the physiologic consequences of the application techniques for various permutations of HFJV is essential to maximize the therapeutic benefit for a given patient and to further define the patients and clinical settings in which HFJV will be most effective.

REFERENCES

1. Drinker, P. and Shaw, L. A., An apparatus for the prolonged administration of artificial respiration. I. A design for adults and children, *J. Clin. Invest.*, 7, 229, 1929.
2. Larsen, H. C. A., Preliminary report on the 1952 epidemic of poliomyelitis in Copenhagen. With special reference to the treatment of acute respiratory insufficiency, *Lancet*, 1, 53, 1953.
3. Sanyal, S. K., Mitchell, C., and Hughes, W. T., Continuous negative chest wall pressure as therapy for severe respiratory distress in older children, *Chest*, 68, 143, 1975.
4. Sanyal, S. K., Bernal, R., and Huges, W. T., Continuous negative chest-wall pressure — successful use for severe respiratory distress in an adult, *JAMA*, 236, 1727, 1976.
5. Holaday, D. A. and Rattenberg, C. C., Automatic lung ventilators, *Anesthesiology*, 23, 493, 1962.
6. Elder, J. D., Jr., et al., An evaluation of mechanical ventilatory devices, *Anesthesiology*, 24, 95, 1963.
7. Ashbaugh, D. G., Bigelow, D. B., and Petty, T. L., Acute respiratory distress in adults, *Lancet*, 2, 319, 1967.
8. Ashbaugh, D. G. and Petty, T. L., Positive end expiratory pressure: physiology, indications and contraindications, *J. Thorac. Cardiovasc. Surg.*, 65, 165, 1973.
9. Sugarman, M. D., Rogers, R. M., and Miller, L. D., Positive end-expiratory pressure (PEEP): indications and physiologic considerations, *Chest*, 62 (Suppl. Part 2), 865, 1972.
10. Kirby, R. R., Robinson, E. J., Schulz, J., et al., A new pediatric volume ventilator. *Anesth. Analg.*, 50, 533, 1971.
11. Downs, J. B., Klein, E. F., Desautels, D., et al., Intermittent mandatory ventilation: a new approach to weaning patients from mechanical ventilators, *Chest*, 64, 331, 1973.
12. Kirby, R. R., Robinson, E. J., Schultz, J., et al., Continuous flow ventilation as an alternative to assisted or controlled ventilation in infants, *Anesth. Analg.*, 51, 871, 1972.
13. Weissman, I. M., Rinaldo, J. E., and Rogers, R. M., State of the Art: intermittent mandatory ventilation, *Am. Rev. Resp. Dis.*, 127, 641, 1983.
14. Shapiro, B. A. and Cane, R. D., The IMV-AMV controversy: a plea for clarification and redirection (editorial), *Crit. Care Med.*, 12, 472, 1984.
15. Kumar, A., Falke, K. I., Geffin, B., et al., Continuous positive pressure ventilation in acute respiratory failure. Effects on hemodynamics and lung function, *N. Engl. J. Med.*, 283, 1430, 1970.
16. Petty, T. and Ashbaugh, D. G., The adult respiratory distress syndrome, *Chest*, 60, 233, 1971.
17. Lutch, J. S. and Murray, J. D., Continuous positive pressure ventilation. Effects on systemic oxygen transport and tissue oxygenation, *Ann. Intern. Med.*, 76, 193, 1972.

18. Falke, K. J., Pontoppidan, H., Kumar, A., et al., Ventilation with end-expiratory pressure in acute lung disease, *J. Clin. Invest.*, 51, 2315, 1972.
19. Pontoppidan, H., Geffin, B., and Lowenstein, E., Acute respiratory failure in the adult, *N. Engl. J. Med.*, 292, 284, 1975.
20. Suter, P. M., et al., Optimum end-expiratory pressure in patients with acute pulmonary failure, *N. Engl. J. Med.*, 292, 284, 1975.
21. Stokke, D. B., Review: artificial ventilation with positive end-expiratory pressure (PEEP), *Eur. J. Intensive Care Med.*, 2, 77, 1976.
22. Ayres, S. M., Mechanisms and consequences of pulmonary edema: cardiac lung, shock lung and principles of ventilatory therapy in adult respiratory distress syndrome, *Am. Heart, J.*, 103, 97, 1982.
23. Balk, R. and Bone, R. C., The adult respiratory distress syndrome, *Med. Clin. N. Am.*, 67, 685, 1983.
24. Brigham, K., Pulmonary edema — cardiac and non-cardiac, *Am. J. Surg.*, 138, 361, 1979.
25. Dantzker, D. R., Brook, C. J., Dehart, P., et al., Ventilation-perfusion disturbances in the adult respiratory distress syndrome, *Am. Rev. Resp. Dis.*, 120, 1039, 1979.
26. Hammon, J. W., Jr., Wolfe, W. G., et al., The effect of positive end-expiratory pressure on regional ventilation and perfusion in the normal and injured primate lung, *J. Thorac. Cardiovas. Surg.*, 72, 680, 1976.
27. Gallagher, T. J., Civetta, J. M., and Kirby, R. R., Terminology update: optimal PEEP, *Crit. Care Med.*, 6, 323, 1978.
28. Gong, H., Positive pressure ventilation in the adult respiratory distress syndrome, *Clin. Chest Med.*, 3, 69, 1982.
29. Kuckelt, W., Scharfenberg, J., Mrochen, H., et al., Effect of PEEP on gas exchange, pulmonary mechanics, and hemodynamics in adult respiratory distress syndrome, *Int. Care Med.*, 7, 177, 1981.
30. Rinaldo, J. E. and Rogers, R. M., Adult respiratory distress syndrome — changing concepts of lung injury and repair, *N. Engl. J. Med.*, 306, 900, 1982.
31. Weissman, I. M., Rinaldo, J. E., and Rogers, R. M., Positive end expiratory pressure in adult respiratory failure, *N. Engl. J. Med.*, 307, 1381, 1982.
32. Shapiro, B. A., Airway pressure therapy for acute restrictive pulmonary pathology, in *Critical Care: State of the Art*, Vol. 2, Shoemaker, W. C. Ed., W. B. Saunders, Philadelphia, 1981.
33. Murray, J. F., Mechanisms of acute respiratory failure, *Am. Rev. Resp. Dis.*, 115, 1071, 1977.
34. Carlon, G. C., Positive end-expiratory pressure: truth and myth, in press.
35. Tyler, D. C., Positive end-expiratory pressure: a review, *Crit. Care Med.*, 11, 300, 1983.
36. Kirby, R. R., Downs, J. B., Civetta, J. M., et al., High level positive end-expiratory pressure (PEEP) in acute respiratory insufficiency, *Chest*, 67, 156, 1975.
37. Kirby, R. R., Perry, J. C., et al., Cardiorespiratory effects of high positive end-expiratory pressure, *Anesthesiology*, 43, 533, 1975.
38. Carter, G. L., Downs, J. B., and Dannemiller, F. J., "Hyper-" end-expiratory pressure in the treatment of adult respiratory insufficiency: a case report, *Anesth. Analg.*, 54, 31, 1975.
39. Kanarek, D. J. and Shannon, D. C., Adverse effect of positive end-expiratory pressure on pulmonary perfusion and arterial oxygenation, *Am. Rev. Resp. Dis.*, 112, 457, 1975.
40. O'Donohue, W. J., Jr., Positive end-expiratory pressure is no panacea (editorial), *Chest*, 76, 373, 1979.
41. Toung, T. J. K., Paharia, P., Mitzner, W. A., et al., The beneficial and harmful effect of positive end-expiratory pressure, *Surg. Gynecol. Obstet.*, 147, 518, 1978.
42. Powers, S. R., Jr., Mannal, R., et al., Physiologic consequences of positive end expiratory pressure (PEEP) ventilation, *Ann. Surg.*, 178, 265, 1973.
43. Springer, R. R. and Stevens, P. M., The influence of PEEP on survival in respiratory failure, *Am. J. Med.*, 66, 196, 1979.
44. Petty, T. L., Why (not) try to PEEP (editorial), *Crit. Care Med.*, 9, 67, 1981.
45. Carlon, G. C., Kahn, R. C., Howland, W. S., et al., Acute life-threatening ventilation-perfusion inequality. An indication for independent lung ventilation, *Crit. Care Med.*, 6, 380, 1978.
46. Carlon, G. C., Ray, C., Klein, R., et al., Criteria for selective positive end-expiratory pressure and independent synchronized ventilation of each lung, *Chest*, 74, 501, 1978.
47. Kveten, V., Carlon, G. C., and Howland, W. S., Acute pulmonary failure in asymmetric lung disease: approach to management, *Crit. Care Med.*, 10, 114, 1982.
48. Gallagher, T. J. and Civetta, J. M., Goal directed therapy of respiratory failure, *Anesth. Analg.*, 59, 831, 1980.
49. Mohsenifar, Z., Golbach, P., et al., Relationship between O_2 delivery and O_2 consumption in the adult respiratory distress syndrome, *Chest*, 84, 267, 1983.
50. Zapol, W. M., Tralstad, R. L., Coffey, J. W., et al., Pulmonary fibrosis in severe acute respiratory failure, *Am. Rev. Resp. Dis.*, 119, 547, 1979.

51. Petty, T. L., What else can injure the lung?, *N. Engl. J. Med.*, 296, 954, 1976.
52. Shoemaker, W. C., Appel, PP., et al., Pathogenesis of respiratory failure (ARDS) after hemorrhage and trauma, *Crit. Care Med.*, 8, 504, 1980.
53. Demling, R. H., The pathogenesis of respiratory failure after trauma and sepsis, *Surg. Clin. North Am.*, 60, 1373, 1980.
54. Pietra, G. G., Ruttner, J. R., et al., The lung after trauma and shock — fine structure of the alveolar-capillary barrier in 23 autopsies, *J. Trauma*, 21, 454, 1981.
55. Brigham, K. L., Mechanisms of lung injury, *Clin. Chest Med.*, 3, 9, 1982.
56. Anderson, R. R., Holliday, R. L., and Driedger, A. A., Documentation of pulmonary capillary permeability in the adult respiratory distress syndrome accompanying human sepsis, *Am. Rev. Resp. Dis.*, 119, 869, 1979.
57. Bell, R. C., Coalson, J. J., et al., Multiple organ system failure and infection in adult respiratory distress syndrome, *Ann. Intern. Med.*, 99, 293, 1983.
58. Fowler, A. A., Hamman, R. F., and Good, J. T., Adult respiratory distress syndrome: risk with common predispositions, *Ann. Intern. Med.*, 99, 593, 1983.
59. Carlon, G. C., Ray, C., Klain, M., et al., High frequency positive pressure ventilation in management of a patient with bronchopleural fistula, *Anesthesiology*, 52, 160, 1980.
60. Carlon, G. C., Howland, W. S., and Groeger, J. S., Early prediction of outcome of respiratory failure, *Chest*, 86, 194, 1980.
61. Carlon, G. C., Respiratory failure in cancer patients, *Curr. Probl. Cancer*, 4, 47, 1979.
62. Caldini, P., Leith, J. D., Brennan, M. J., Effect of continuous positive-pressure ventilation (CPPV) on edema formation in dog lung, *J. Appl. Physiol.*, 39, 672, 1975.
63. Demling, R. H., Staub, N. C., and Edmunds, L. H., Effect of end-expiratory airway pressure on accumulation of extravascular water, *J. Appl. Physiol.*, 38, 905, 1975.
64. Hopewell, P. C. and Murray, J. F., Effects of continuous positive pressure ventilation in experimental pulmonary edema, *J. Appl. Physiol.*, 40, 568, 1976.
65. Hopewell, P. C., Failure of positive end-expiratory pressure to decrease lung water in alloxan induced pulmonary edema, *Am. Rev. Resp. Dis.*, 120, 813, 1979.
66. Wyszogrodski, I., Kyei-Aboagye, K., Taeusch, H., Jr., et al., Surfactant inactivation by hyperventilation: conservation by end-expiratory pressure, *J. Appl. Physiol.*, 38, 461, 1975.
67. Zapol, W. M., Snider, M. T., and Schneider, R. C., Extracorporeal membrane oxygenation for acute respiratory insufficiency, *Anesthesiology*, 46, 272, 1977.
68. National Heart Lung and Blood Institute, Division of Lung Disease, Extracorporeal Support for Respiratory Insufficiency, National Institutes of Health, Bethesda, Md, 1979, 243.
69. Pierce, E. C., Is extracorporeal membrane oxygenation a viable technique?, *Ann. Thorac. Surg.*, 31, 102, 1980.
70. Henderson, Y., Chillingworth, F. D., and Whitney, J. L., The respiratory dead space, *Am. J. Physiol.*, 38, 1, 1915.
71. Bjerager, K., Sjostrand, U., and Wattwil, M., Long-term treatment of two patients with respiratory insufficiency with IPPV/PEEP and HFPPV/PEEP, *Acta Anesth. Scand.*, Suppl. 64, 55, 1977.
72. Jonzon, A., Sedin, G., Oberg, P. A., and Sjostrand, U., High-frequency positive-pressure ventilation by endotracheal insufflation, *Acta Anaesth. Scand.*, Suppl. 43, 1, 1971.
73. Sjostrand, U., Review of the physiological rationale for and development of high-frequency positive-pressure ventilation — HFPPV, *Acta Anaesth. Scand.*, Suppl. 64, 7, 1977.
74. Bunegin, L., Borg, U. R., Helsel, P., et al., Cerebral blood flow during HFPPV and IPPV at normal and elevated ICP, *Anesthesiology*, 57, A465, 1982.
75. El-Baz, N., El-Ganzouri, et al., One-lung high-frequency positive-pressure ventilation for sleeve pneumonectomy: an alternative technique, *Anesth. Analg.*, 60, 683, 1981.
76. Eriksson, I., The role of the conducting airways in gas exchange during high frequency ventilation — a clinical and theoretical analysis, *Anesth. Analg.*, 61, 483, 1982.
77. Jonzon, A., Phrenic and vagal nerve activities during spontaneous and positive pressure ventilation, *Acta Anaesth. Scand.*, Suppl. 64, 29, 1977.
78. Malina, J. R., Nordstrom, S. G., Sjostrand, U., et al., Clinical evaluation of high-frequency ventilation (HFPPV) in patients scheduled for open-chest surgery, *Anesth. Analg.*, 60, 234, 1981.
79. Sjostrand, U., Ed., Experimental and clinical evaluation of high-frequency positive-pressure ventilation — HFPPV (editorial), *Acta Anaesth. Scand.*, Suppl. 64, 5, 1977.
80. Wattwil, L. M., Evaluation of HFPPV in experimental and clinical practice, *Acta Univ. Ups.*, 416, 1982.
81. Wattwil, L. M., Sjostrand, U. H., and Borg, U. R., Comparative studies of IPPV and HFPPV with PEEP in critical care patients — a clinical evaluation, *Crit. Care Med.*, 11, 30, 1983.
82. Wattwil, L. M., Sjostrand, U. H., Borg, U. R., and Eriksson, I. A., Comparative studies of IPPV and HFPPV with PEEP in critical care patients — studies on intrapulmonary gas distribution, *Crit. Care Med.*, 11, 38, 1983.

83. Sutton, J. E. and Glass, D. D., Airway pressure gradient during high-frequency ventilation, *Crit. Care Med.*, 12, 774, 1983.
84. Pinchak, A. C., Hagen, J. F., and Hancock, D., et al., High frequency positive pressure ventilation with the MA-1 ventilator, *Crit. Care Med.*, 12, 810, 1984.
85. Smith, R. B. and Sjostrand, U. H., Eds., High frequency ventilation, *Int. Anesth. Clin.*, 21, 3, 1983.
86. Scheck, P. A., Sjostrand, U. H., and Smith, R. B., Eds., *Perspectives in High Frequency Ventilation*, Martinus Nijhoff, Boston, 1983.
87. Sjostrand, U. H., High-frequency positive-pressure ventilation (HFPPV): a review, *Crit. Care Med.*, 8, 345, 1980.
88. Borg, U., Eriksson, I., and Sjostrand, U. H., High-frequency positive pressure ventilation (HFPPV): a review based upon its use during bronchoscopy and for laryngoscopy and microlaryngeal surgery under general anesthesia, *Anesth. Analg.*, 59, 594, 1980.
89. Kirby, R. R., High-frequency positive-pressure ventilation (HFPPV): what role in ventilatory insufficiency?, *Anesthesiology*, 52, 109, 1980.
90. Howland, W. S. and Carlon, G. C., Development of high-frequency ventilation techniques, *Crit. Care Med.*, 12, 705, 1984.
91. Scheck, P. A., High frequency positive pressure ventilation: utilization in the operating room, in press.
92. Gettinger, A. and Glass, D. D., HFPPV: use in neonatal and adult intensive care, in press.
93. Jacoby, J. J., Hamelburg, W., Ziegler, C. H., et al., Transtracheal resuscitation, *JAMA*, 162, 625, 1956.
94. Sanders, R. D., Two ventilating attachments for bronchoscopes, *Del. Med. J.*, 39, 170, 1967.
95. Rock, J. J., Pfaeffle, H., Smith, R. B., Klain, M., et al., High pressure jet insufflation used to prevent aspiration and its effect on the tracheal mucosal wall, *Crit. Care Med.*, 4, 134, 1976.
96. Smith, R. B. and Klain, M., High frequency percutaneous transtracheal jet ventilation, *Crit. Care Med.*, 5, 280, 1977.
97. Klain, M. and Smith, R. B., Fluidic technology, *Anesthesia*, 31, 750, 1976.
98. Calkins, J. M., Waterson, C. K., Hammeroff, S. R., et al., A simple fleuric high frequency jet ventilator, *Anesth. Analg.*, 61, 138, 1982.
99. Smith, R. B. and Klain, M., Experimental high frequency jet ventilation, *Int. Anesth. Clin.*, 21, 33, 1983.
100. Carlon, G. C., Miodownik, S., Ray, C., Jr., and Kahn, R. C., Technical aspects and clinical implication of high frequency jet ventilation with a solenoid valve, *Crit. Care Med.*, 9, 47, 1981.
101. Carlon, G. C., Miodownik, S., and Ray, C., Jr., Characterization of high frequency ventilators, in press.
102. Miodownik, S., High-frequency jet ventilation: technical implications, *Crit. Care Med.*, 12, 718, 1984.
103. Groeger, J. S., Carlon, G. C., Howland, W. S., et al., Experimental evaluation of high-frequency jet ventilation, *Crit. Care Med.*, 12, 747, 1981.
104. Carlon, G. C., Ray, C., Jr., Groeger, J. S., et al., Tidal volume and airway pressure on high frequency jet ventilation, *Crit. Care Med.*, 1, 83, 1983.
105. Calkins, J. M., High frequency jet ventilation: experimental evaluation, in press.
106. Carlon, G. C., Ray, C., Jr., Miodownik, S., Howland, W. S., et al., Physiologic implications of high frequency jet ventilation techniques, *Crit. Care Med.*, 11, 508, 1983.
107. Scacci, R., Air entrainment masks — jet mixing is how they work — the Bernouli and Venturi principles is how they don't, *Resp. Care*, 24, 298, 1979.
108. Robinson, J. L., *Basic Fluid Mechanics*, McGraw-Hill, New York, 1963, 85.
109. Nunn, J. F., *Applied Respiratory Physiology*, 2nd ed., Butterworth, London, 1977, 96.
110. Carlon, G. C., Ray, C., Jr., Goetz, W. S., and Groeger, J. S., High frequency jet ventilation in respiratory failure: influence of drining pressure and cannula size, *Crit. Care Med.*, 9(Abstrs), 159, 1981.
111. Carlon, G. C., Ray, C., Jr., Miodownik, S., and Kaczmarck, M. E., Bench Evaluation of High Frequency Jet Ventilation, 19th Annual Meeting of the Association for the Advancement of Medical Instrumentation, Washington, D.C., April 15—18, 1984.
112. Rolly, G. and Versichele, L., Gas analysis by mass spectrometry during high frequency ventilation, in *Perspectives in High Frequency Ventilation*, Scheck, P. A., Sjostrand, U. H., Smith, R. B., Eds., Martinus Nijhoff, Boston, 1983, 164.
113. Calkins, J. M., Waterson, C. K., Hammeroff, S. R., and Kaner, J., Jet pulse characteristics for high frequency jet ventilation in dogs, *Anesth. Analg.*, 61, 293, 1982.
114. Davey, A. J., Lay, G. R., and Leigh, J. M., High frequency venturi jet ventilation: comparison of a proximal central jet with a distal wall jet, *Anesthesiology*, 37, 947, 1982.

115. Woo, P. S., Eurenius. Dynamics of venturi jet ventilation through the operating laryngoscope, *Ann. Otol. Rhinol. Laryngol.*, 91, 615, 1982.
116. Davey, A. J., Lay, G. R., and Leigh, J. M., High frequency venturi jet ventilation: a functional analysis of the Penlon Nuffield Series 200 Ventilator, *Anesthesiology*, 37, 675, 1982.
117. Lyons, D., Stenzler, A., Steinberg, H., et al., The airway mechanics of jet ventilation, *Otolaryngol, Head Neck Surg.*, 89, 364, 1981.
118. Beamer, W. C., Prough, D. S., Royster, R. L., et al., High Frequency Jet Ventilation Produces Auto-PEEP, Proc. Int. Symp. High Frequency Ventilation, Memorial Sloan-Kettering Cancer Center 1983, p. 63—66.
119. Babinski, M. F., Bunegin, L., Smith, R. B., and Hoff, B. H., Application of double lumen tracheal tubes for HFV, *Anesthesiology*, Suppl. 55, 370, 1981.
120. Waterson, C. K., Militzer, H. W., Quan, S. F., and Calkins, J. M., Airway pressure as a measure of gas exchange during high frequency jet ventilation, *Crit. Care Med.*, 12, 742, 1984.
121. Ray, C., Jr., Theroetical Basis for High Frequency Jet Ventilation, Proc. Int. Symp. High Frequency Ventilation, Memorial Sloan-Kettering Cancer Center, 1983, p. 9—11.
122. Carlon, G. C., Ray, C., Jr., Klain, M., and McCormack, P. M., High frequency positive pressure ventilation in management of a patient with bronchopleural fistula, *Anesthesiology*, 52, 160, 1980.
123. Turnbull, A. D., Carlon, G. C., Howland, W. S., and Beattie, E. J., Jr., High frequency jet ventilation in major airway or pulmonary disruption, *Ann. Thorac. Surg.*, 32, 468, 1981.
124. Carlon, G. C., Kahn, R. C., Howland, W. S., Ray, C., Jr., and Turnbull, A. D., Clinical experience with high frequency jet ventilation, *Crit. Care Med.*, 9, 1, 1981.
125. Carlon, G. C., Ray, C., Jr., Pierri, M. K., Groeger, J. S., and Howland, W. S., High frequency jet ventilation. Theoretical considerations and clinical observations, *Chest*, 81, 350, 1982.
126. Carlon, G. C., Griffin, J., Ray, C., Jr., Groeger, J. S., and Patrick, K., High frequency jet ventilation in experimental airway disruption, *Crit. Care Med.*, 11, 353, 1983.
127. Smith, R. B., Hoff, B. H., Bennett, E. V., Wilson, E. A., Grover, F. L., Babinski, M. F., and Sjostrand, U. H., High frequency ventilation and IPPV in the presence of a bronchopleural fistula, in *Perspectives in High Frequency Ventilation*, Martinus Nijhoff, Boston, 1983, 316.
128. Smith, R. B. and Babinski, M. F., Clinical high frequency jet ventilation, *Int. Anesth. Clin.*, 21, 89, 1983.
129. Benjaminsson, E. and Klain, M., Intraoperative dual mode independent lung ventilation of a patient with bronchopleural fistula, *Anesth. Analg.*, 60, 118, 1981.
130. Derderian, S. S., Rajagopal, K. R., Abbrecht, P. H., Bennett, L. L., Doblar, D. D., and Hunt, K. K., High frequency positive pressure jet ventilation in bilateral bronchopleural fistula, *Crit. Care Med.*, 10, 119, 1982.
131. Carlon, G. C. and Howland, W. S., Clinical experience with high frequency jet ventilation, *Int. Anesth. Clin.*, 21, 99, 1983.
132. El-Baz, N., El-Ganzouri, A., and Ivankovich, A., High frequency positive pressure ventilation for major airway surgery, in *Perspectives in High Frequency Ventilation*, Martinus Nijhoff, Boston, 1983, 216.
133. Carlon, G. C., Turnbull, A. D., Alexander, J. D., Howland, W. S., and Beattie, E. J., *Crit. Care Med.*, 9, 163, 1981.
134. Nunn, J. F., *Applied Respiratory Physiology*, 2nd ed, Butterworth, London, 1977, 94.
135. Versprille, A., A simple mathematical model of high frequency ventilation, in *Perspectives in High Frequency Ventilation*, Martinus Nijhoff, Boston, 1983, 1.
136. Slutsky, A. S., Kamm, R. D., and Drazen, J. M., High frequency oscillatory ventilation using tidal volumes smaller than anatomical dead space, *Int. Anesth. Clin.*, 21, 161, 1983.
137. Slutsky, A. S., Kamm, R. D., and Drazen, J. M., A review of theoretical and experimental studies of high frequency ventilation, in *Perspectives in High Frequency Ventilation*, Martinus Nijhoff, Boston, 1983, 59.
138. Rossing, T. H., Slutsky, A. S., Lehr, J. L., Drinker, P. A., Kamm, R., and Drazen, J. M., Tidal volume and frequency dependence of carbon dixoide elimination by high frequency ventilation, *N. Engl. J. Med.*, 305, 1375, 1981.
139. Carlon, G. C., Howland, W. S., Ray, C., Miodownik, S., Griffin, J. P., and Groeger, J. S., High frequency jet ventilation. A prospective randomized evaluation, *Chest*, 84, 551, 1983.
140. Bourgain, J. L., Mortimer, A. J., and Sykes, M. K., Carbon dixoide clearance during high frequency jet ventilation (HFJV), in *Perspective in High Frequency Ventilation*, Martinus Nijhoff, Boston, 1983, 98.
141. Slustky, A. S., Mechanisms affecting gas transport during high frequency oscillation, *Crit. Care Med.*, 12, 713, 1984.
142. Jaeger, M. J., Kurzweg, U., and Banner, M. J., Transport of gases in high-frequency ventilation, *Crit. Care Med.*, 12, 708, 1984.

143. Fredberg, J. J., Augmented diffusion in the airways can support pulmonary gas exchange, *J. Appl. Physiol.*, 49, 232, 1980.

144. Calkins, J. M., Waterson, C. K., Quan, S. F., Militzer, H. W., Conahan, T. J., Otto, C. W., and Hameroff, S. R., Effects of high frequency jet ventilation design and operational variables upon arterial blood gas tensions, in *Perspectives in High Frequency Ventilation*, Martinus Nijhoff, Boston, 1983, 71.

145. Fletcher, P. R., Alveolar pressures during high frequency ventilation, in *Perspectives in High Frequency Ventilation*, Martinus Nijhoff, Boston, 1983, 92.

146. Klain, M., Gas exchange in high frequency ventilation: an experimental study, in *Perspectives in High Frequency Ventilation*, Martinus Nijhoff, Boston, 1983, 158.

147. Ray, C., Jr., Miodownik, S., Carlon, G. C., Groeger, J. S., and Howland, U. S., Pneumatic-to-electrical analog model of the high frequency jet ventilation of disrupted airways, *Crit. Care Med.*, 12, 711, 1984.

148. Pierson, D. J., Persistent bronchopleural air leak during mechanical ventilation: a review, *Respir. Care*, 27, 408, 1982.

149. Petty, T. L., Adult respiratory distress syndrome: definition and historical perspective, *Clin. Chest Med.*, 3, 3, 1982.

Chapter 10

HIGH FREQUENCY VENTILATION IN THE OPERATING ROOM

Jerry M. Calkins

TABLE OF CONTENTS

I. INTRODUCTION

The successful use of HFV in the operating room (OR) depends upon an understanding of the design principles and performance characteristics of the ventilator. Prior clinical applications have established the safety and efficacy of HFV. However, the choice to use HFV is influenced by the physical status of the patient, potential physiologic advantages and disadvantages, the requirements of the surgical situation, and the ability to adequately oxygenate and ventilate with each technique.

II. TECHNIQUES OF DELIVERING HFV IN THE OR

HFV is a method of ventilatory support which can achieve effective alveolar ventilation and oxygenation at frequencies between 60 and 2400 c/min. It is usually associated with low airway pressures and tidal volumes less than or equivalent to the anatomic dead space volume.[1,2]

The three most common techniques of delivering HFV are HFPPV, HFJV, and HFOV.[1,2] HFPPV employs a constant volume ventilator with a small compressible volume at frequencies up to 100 cycles/min (1.7 Hz).[3,4] HFJV utilizes the pulsation of a small jet of gas introduced into the airway via a catheter located either directly within the trachea or within an endotracheal tube.[5-7] The gas flow is generated from a regulated high pressure source and usually controlled by either a fluidic or electromechanical control system. This technique is effective at ventilatory frequencies ranging from 60 to 900 c/min (1—5 Hz). In HFOV, pressure oscillations are superimposed upon a steady bias gas flow. The bias flow provides fresh gas to the breathing circuit.[8,9] HFOV has been studied at frequencies ranging from 120 to 2400/min (2—40 Hz).

Within these major categories, variations of delivery technique have been investigated. For example a fluidic high frequency jet ventilator has been utilized to provide high frequency alternating lung ventilation (HFALV).[10] With HFALV, each lung is ventilated by HFJV independently and 180° out of phase with the other. The potential clinical benefits of HFALV have not been completely determined.

In spite of the mechanical differences among the three major categories of HFV delivery methods, all share some common characteristics. First, effective gas exchange occurs at ventilatory frequencies higher than those of CMV or spontaneous breathing. Second, peak airway pressures are lower than those observed with CMV. Third, ventilation occurs with tidal volume close to or less than the anatomic dead space volume.

The exact mechanisms of gas transport with HFV are unclear. However, effective gas exchange with HFV has been demonstrated in numerous acute care situations. These applications include emergency airway management during cardiopulmonary resuscitation, anesthesia and surgical procedures, and ventilatory support of critically ill pediatric and adult patients.[11] The preponderance of study and utilization of HFV in the operating room has emphasized the use of HFPPV and HFJV.[12] Limited data on the use of HFOV in this setting is beginning to be reported.[13]

At this time, no mode of HFV has demonstrated a significant advantage over CMV for routine respiratory support in the operating room. Nonetheless, potential advantages theoretically exist in applying HFV in the clinical situation. This chapter explores the physiologic aspects of HFV influencing its selection for OR applications and discusses the anesthetic/surgical situations where it has been successfully applied.

III. PHYSIOLOGIC CONSIDERATIONS FOR HFV APPLICATIONS IN THE OR

In general the physiologic effects of HFV result directly from using lower peak airway pressures, higher ventilatory frequencies, and smaller tidal volumes (usually less than anatomic dead space volume). At equivalent ventilatory conditions, peak intratracheal pressures are substantially lower with HFV than with IPPV. A lower intratracheal pressure should produce a corresponding lower intrathoracic pressure. Hence, HFV should decrease the incidence of barotrauma.

Although interactions between chest expansion and pulmonary hemodynamic variables have been noted, no significant harmful effects of either HFPPV or HFJV on either the pathology or physiology of the lung tissue and tracheal mucosa, have been observed.[14-16] The adverse effects observed may be secondary to inadequate preconditioning of the ventilatory gases and techniques used to introduce the catheter into the airway. As with CMV, inadequate humidification of gases delivered by HFJV impairs mucociliary transport, while adequate humidification preserves it.[17] Percutaneous transtracheal jet ventilation has been associated with increased incidence of tracheal mucosal damage, subcutaneous emphysema, pneudomediastium, and pneumopericardium.[18]

One major concern in the OR is protection of the airway from aspiration. Investigations have been conducted to assess airway protection in situations where an HFJV insufflation catheter was used without an endotracheal tube. In a series of studies, Klain et al. considered the effects of frequency and I:E ratio on aspiration during CPR in dogs.[19] Without chest compression, no aspiration occurred if expiration was no longer than 66% of the cycle (I:E = 1:2) or if frequency was greater than 60 c/min (1 Hz).[20] With chest compressions, no evidence of aspiration occurred if expiration was not more than 50% of the cycle (I:E = 1:1) and frequency was at least 100 c/min (1.7 Hz). In a third series using the same technique, an upper airway obstruction was created using a radio opaque food stuff. Transtracheal HFJV was evaluated in removing the obstruction as a Heimlich type mancuver.[20] The process was assessed by radionematography. Material above the jet tended to be expelled into the mouth. Material below the jet was propelled deeper into the lungs. Szele and Keenan demonstrated that once percutaneous transtracheal HFJV is begun at 150 c/min (2.5 Hz), 30% inspiratory time (30% I time = I:E of 3:7), and MAP of 4 torr, aspiration may be prevented if the oropharynx if free of foreign material. If material is present before HFJV is begun, care must be taken to properly direct the jet catheter.[21]

The potential adverse cardiovascular effects of conventional mechanical ventilation are related to positive airway and intrapleural pressures which may impair venous return to the right heart and decrease cardiac output. By contrast, HFV may be expected to interfere less with venous return and hence cause less hemodynamic impairment. This is due to its reduced peak and possibly lower MAP. HFV have reported enhanced, reduced, and unchanged hemodynamic function compared to conventional ventilation (Table 1).[4,22-34] Synchronization of ventilation with the cardiac cycle during HFJV might actually augment circulation and hence increase cardiac output.[16] Data from one set of limited animal studies suggested that cardiac output was significantly lower with IPPV than with HFPPV.[4] This difference disappeared when HFJV was compared to IPPV in healthy dogs.[17] However, with the addition of 15 cm H_2O of PEEP, cardiac output during HFJV was greater than with CMV and PEEP. Synchronizing the high frequency pulse with the ECG did not increase cardiac output over unsynchronized HFJV. Eosphageal echocardiography has been used to further assess left ventricular function during HFJV and IPPV in anesthetized patients undergoing low abdominal surgery.[15,37] No significant change in function was noted between modes. The results of these studies suggest that HFV may be useful when IPPV would produce an unacceptable decrease in cardiac output. Unfortunately, the cardiovascular effects of HFV and IPPV have not been compared in patients with parenchymal disease.

IPPV produces cyclic changes in intrathoracic pressure which produce large fluctua-

Table 1
HEMODYNAMIC EFFECTS OF HFV

Subjects	Type of HFV	P_{AW} HFV	Hemodynamic effect of HFV	Ref.
Dogs	HFPPV	Lower	++	29
Patients	HFO	?	=	9
Patients	HFJV	?	=	26
Patients	HFJV	?	= or ++	5
Patients	HFJV	Higher	=	25
Dogs	Emerson	?	−−	28
Dogs	HFJV	Lower	=	21, 30
Dogs	HFJV	Higher	−−	5, 31
Dogs	HFJV	Lower	++	23
Patients	HFJV	Lower	=	11, 32
Dogs	HFJV	Lower	++	33
Patients	HFJV	?	=	34

Note: (++) improved, (=) unchanged, (−−) impaired.

tions in ICP. These fluctuations are clearly reduced during HFPPV and HFJV. The physical movement of the brain is likewise less pronounced.[35-37] However, mean ICP does not decrease with either HFPPV or HFJV, and there is little effect on cerebral hemodynamics.[35,38] Babinski et al.[39] demonstrated that ICP fluctuations were less in normocarbic dogs with HFJV at 100 to 150 c/min (1.7—2.5 Hz) than at lower frequencies. This has also been demonstrated in dogs with intracranial hypertension. Absolute values of mean ICP in these groups of animals were not affected by HFJV, and brain movement was reduced. In another study, no significant cerebral lesions were observed by gross and histologic examination in 12 mongrel dogs supported on HFJV and IPPV for 4 hr.[15]

Another potential advantage of HFV is the rapidity with which air embolisms are cleared from the pulmonary vasculature. Hoff et al.[40] compared the effects of IPPV and HFOV at 1200 c/min (20 Hz) in healthy dogs with the rapid intravenous infusion of 6.6 mℓ/kg of an air/xenon mixture. In animals which did not develop an air lock, HFOV resulted in a more rapid clearance of the embolized gases from the right ventricle and lungs. When an air lock developed, cardiovascular collapse occurred with demise of the animal, regardless of the mode of ventilation. It is unclear, however, whether clinical studies will confirm the potential usefulness of HFV in neurosurgery.

During conventional IPPV, glomerular filtration rate (GFR), urine volume, and urine sodium excretion decrease. These changes have been attributed to a decreased cardiac output, a secondary increase in sympathetic tone with a resultant stimulation of the renin-angiotensin system, increased antidiuretic hormone (ADH) secretion, and reduced free water clearance. More recently, alterations in renal vein pressures and renal pulsatile flow patterns, induced by IPPV, have been implicated.[41] Results from limited studies indicate that HFPPV does not produce a similar renal effect.[42] The absence of ADH hypersecretion may be related to lower intrathoracic pressures. When HFPPV is utilized in experimental animals, free water clearance is normal and water loads are excreted without delay.[42] Marquez et al. compared renal function in swine with HFJV at 100 c/min (1.7 Hz) an I:E ratio of 0.3, and a 10 cm H_2O PEEP or 10 cm H_2O CPAP to spontaneously ventilating animals.[41] Their preliminary results indicate that neither of the airway pressure patterns altered GFR or venous renin. Urine volume was decreased with both ventilatory modes, but urine sodium excretion was decreased only during HFJV with PEEP.

Table 2
CLINICAL EXPERIENCE WITH HFJV AT ARIZONA HEALTH SCIENCES CENTER

Category of procedure	No. studied	Age range	Frequencies studied (min^{-1})	% Inspiratory time studied	Duration on HFJV (min)
General					
Upper abdominal[a]	6	23—80	150—600	20—30	18—325
Lower abdominal[b]	31	22—71	150—450	10—50	17—244
Orthopedic Extremity	9	60—72	150—300	10—30	15—60
General/plastic	2	52—67	150—300	10—30	15—30
Thoracic	3	29—76	60—300	10—30	15—60
Neurosurgical					
Craniotomy	7	16—58	60—300	10—30	15—90
Spinal[c]	3	41—52	150—300	10—30	15—90
Vascular	2	56—62	150—300	10—30	30—120

[a] Primarily laparotomy or cholecystectomy.
[b] Primarily abdominal hysterectomy or ovarian surgery.
[c] Primarily cervical fusion; hypercarbia observed in one patient.

Table 3
ABG'S DURING OPERATING ROOM APPLICATIONS OF HFJV

Applications	Patients	ABG[a]		
		PO_2	PCO_2	PH
Oral surgery	100	455	32	7.44
Laryngoscopy/bronchoscopy	11	359	42	7.34
Thoracic/cardiac	14	298	40	7.37
Abdominal surgery	52	290	33	7.43
Plastic/orthopedic	36	370	32	7.45

[a] PO_2, PCO_2 – mm Hg

This effort was extended to an assessment of renal function and renin secretion in postsurgical patients during HFJV with airway pressures at either zero end expiratory pressure (ZEEP) or 10 cm H_2O PEEP. HFJV with ZEEP maintained normal renal and cardiovascular function. Urinary flow and GFR was normal, with a spontaneous solute natriuresis. However, when HFJV with PEEP was utilized, both cardiovascular and renal function deteriorated. Urinary flow and GFR decreased, resulting in a diminished free water clearance and sodium retention.

IV. APPLICATIONS IN THE OR

HFV has been successfully utilized during anesthesia in a variety of surgical procedures (Tables 2 and 3).[12,44] The preponderance of OR applications has been with HFPPV and HFJV. There is limited experience utilizing HFOV clinically.[13] HFJV and HFPPV have been used in various surgical procedures where surgeons and anesthesiologists are competing for the same space as in laser microsurgery of the larynx, bronchoscopy, laryngoscopy, sleeve pneumonectomies, and tracheal reconstruction. HFV appears to be useful during other ENT, orthopedic general, thoracic, and neurosurgical procedures.

A. Upper Airway Procedures

HFPPV and HFJV have been used extensively in the OR for ventilation during rigid bronchoscopy, laryngoscopy, and microscopic laryngeal laser surgery.[4,7,45-50] In these situation, the surgeon and the anesthesiologist compete for the patient's airway. Special ventilation techniques are necessary.[69] Repeated interruption of the surgical procedure was usually necessary to maintain adequate ventilation.

Prior to the acceptance of conventional jet ventilation (CJV-Sanders technique), spontaneous ventilation and apenic insufflation techniques were employed.[52-54] However, the advent of CJV was a significant advance for ventilating patients during bronchoscopy and laryngoscopy. Improved CJV has now been followed by the further development of HFPPV and HFJV. Either CJV or HFV have proven to be satisfactory. Current trends are to use CJV in instances where an endotracheal tube (ETT) is not utilized, while HFV may be employed with or without an ETT.

When no ETT is used, one disadvantage of jet ventilation is air entrainment, which causes a room air dilution of gas delivered by the ventilator. The degree to which this occurs depends primarily on the gas-flow rates used, jet orifice design, and the effective trachea diameter.[71] High flow rates and a decreased jet-diameter to trachea-diameter ratio leads to the greatest degree of air entrainment. Because of air entrainment, the patient potentially may receive less than 100% oxygen, leading to hypoventilation and development of hypoxemia and hypercarbia. However, Ruder et al.[70] measured arterial blood gas tensions (ABG) preoperatively and intraoperatively in patients undergoing microlaryngeal surgery with jet ventilation. These results indicated the patients were adequately ventilated without hypercarbia or hypoxemia. Although oxygen and nitrous oxide have been used, it is not possible to deliver a volatile anesthetic gas mixture. In addition, there is a risk of barotrauma from the high airway pressures with the jet technique.

With HFPPV, the anesthetist can administer high oxygen concentrations and deliver an anesthetic gas mixture via the sidearm of the bronchoscope. This is feasible because unlike the injector technique there is no gas entrainment during HFPPV ventilation.[12]

With laryngoscopy, a translaryngeal, nasotracheal, or orotracheal insufflation catheter is inserted. Side holes near the catheter tip and an outwardly directed flow of gas through the larynx prevent the entrainment of room air.

In addition to this problem, air entrainment may force laser induced smoke, particulate material and/or blood into the lungs. In order to minimize this problem, gas injection during CJV inspiration is not recommended at the moment the laser is employed. This is more difficult to accomplish with HFV.[69]

If the distal tip of the catheter is inadvertently placed proximal to the vocal cords, insufflation of the stomach may occur. This increased the potential for gastric distension and regurgitation. A nasogastric tube may be employed to remove stomach contents and gas if necessary. Another problem with a misplaced catheter tip is tracheal perforation. Both of these potential problems are minimized by proper positioning of the catheter and utilization of an adequate supply gas pressure.

B. Thoracic Surgery

The possibility of HFJV application for ventilatory support during thoracic surgical procedures and experimental airway disruptions has also been investigated.[57-68] Hoff et al.[57] compared percutaneous transtracheal HFJV with IPPV in healthy dogs before and after thoracotomy. Adequate gas exchange at low MAP was obtained at frequencies of 100 (1.7 Hz) and 300 c/min (5 Hz) with IPPV. The lowest PaO_2 and $PaCO_2$ occurred at 100 c/min (1.7 Hz). In addition, the chest was more quiescent during HFJV. Carlon et al.[58] demonstrated that HFJV can provide effective ventilation with air leaks through various openings.

The administration of gases via the jet method has been effective in major airway surgery.[59,60,65,67] During sleeve pneumonectomies and tracheal reconstruction, it may be difficult to provide adequate ventilation without impairing access to the surgical field. To circumvent this problem, a small bore catheter is inserted into the distal bronchus or trachea when the airway is transected. Effective ventilation can then be delivered via this catheter using HFJV.

The use of another technique, HFALV has been suggested for thoracic surgery.[10] With this technique, bronchial catheters are placed in each main stem bronchus. Jet ventilation is then delivered to each catheter independently in one of several combinations. These combinations include both jets pulsed together at either low or high frequency; the jets pulsed alternately, 180° out of phase (HFALV); or the jets pulsed asynchronously. A lower $PaCO_2$ and arterial-alveolar oxygen gradient was obtained with HFALV than HFJV.

C. Neurosurgery

Potential clinical applications exist for HFV in neurosurgical procedures.[35-40] As previously discussed, the significant decrease in cerebral motion and ICP fluctuation, without cerebral hemodynamic changes, may offer advantages to the neurosurgeon. Air embolism is also often a serious problem during craniotomies and preliminary data suggest that HFJV may facilitate dissolution of air emboli within the pulmonary vasculature.

D. Urological Surgery

Extracorporeal shock wave lithotripsy (ESWL) is becoming widely accepted as an important therapeutic regime for nephrolithiasis. The efficiency of ESWL comes from maintaining a precise unchanging location of the renal stone. Stability of the stone position assists in focusing the shock waves which results in a reduction of both wave intensity and the number of repetitions.[73-75]

During either spontaneous or conventional mechanical ventilation, significant lung-thorax and diaphragmatic movement occurs. Diaphragmatic displacement, in turn, produces abdominal excursions which move both stone and healthy tissue into and out of the ESWL focus. Since the lower peak inspiratory pressure of HFJV tends to minimize lung-thorax and diaphragmatic motion during inhalation, abdominal movement is also reduced. With smaller abdominal excursions, the renal stone is more stationary during HFJV.[74,75] This results in a reduction of impulses at a lower intensity as well as a shortened length of procedure time.[74,75]

E. Other Surgical Procedures

HFJV and HFPPV have been employed effectively in a large number of orthopedic, abdominal, and spinal surgical procedures.[12,15,44] For example, in nearly every case at the Arizona Health Sciences Center (Table 2), adequate gas exchange was observed. There have been no significant problems with hypotension, arrhythmias, or barotrauma. Although a ventilatory frequency of 150 c/min (2.5 Hz) and an inspiratory time of 30% was used in most patients, higher frequencies and different inspiratory times have been evaluated in a few cases. Frequencies greater than 300/min (5 Hz) generally resulted in carbon dioxide retention, even with adjustments in the inspiratory time and airway pressure. Furthermore, an airway pressure excursion (Peak-PEEP) of at least 3 cm H_2O appears to be necessary to assure adequate CO_2 elimination. Although effective ventilation could be provided using high frequency techniques during these surgical procedures, a clear advantage over conventional mechanical ventilation was not demonstrated. Without specific, demonstrable benefit, the role of HFV in routine elective surgical procedures remains to be defined.

V. HFV IN THE OR: POTENTIAL CONCERNS

Several major concerns regarding the use of HFV in the operating room are centered on assuring and assessing adequate gas exchange while preventing barotrauma. The effective tidal volume during HFV, unlike with a constant volume ventilator, is not determined solely by volume output of the ventilator. The characteristics of the patient's respiratory system can also affect the delivered volume. Therefore, any action that increases respiratory system impedance may diminish the effectiveness of ventilation during HFV. For example, if a member of the surgical team leans on the patient's chest or if upward retraction is applied against the diaphragm, ventilation may be adversely affected.

A rough estimate of the adequacy of ventilation may be obtained by observing chest-wall excursions. Even with a rapid ventilatory rate, there should be visible movement of the thoracic chest. Lack of motion is evidence of hypoventilation, which must be immediately corrected. As with CMV, precise evaluation of gas exchange requires ABG analysis. Unlike CMV, standard ventilator settings which results in adequate ABG tensions with HFJV have not been completely defined. Hence, ABGs, are essential soon after initiating HFJV, and after any actions which may affect ventilation efficiency.

Another concern is the prevention of barotrauma and cardiac compromise. The pressure required to introduce each jet pulse may be as high as 50 psi. Inadvertent impedance to exhalation during rapid gas pulsations can overpressurize the airway, which may result in pneumothorax or severe cardiac compromise. Hence, airway pressure monitoring is essential.[11]

Other disadvantages of jet ventilation through a catheter include tracheal barotrauma, gas dissection along the tracheal mucosa, and pneumothorax. All of these complications are related to the delivery pressure of the jet gas and may be avoided with proper selection of source gas pressure. It is essential to start with low gas supply pressures and increase slowly to the appropriate level. Airway pressure should be monitored in order to prevent these complications. Increased airway resistance secondary to large laryngeal lesions, tracheal stenosis, bronchoscopic examination, and poor lung compliance may prevent the outflow of injected gas, thereby increasing the potential for tissue dissection, barotrauma, and pneumothroax. The incidence of a pneumothorax significant enough to require chest tube placement has been reported to be approximately 1%.[70]

As previously discussed, other concerns include protection of the airway when only a catheter is used, and dilution secondary to entrainment. The effects of frequency and I/E ratio on the prevention of aspiration have been investigated and, under certain conditions, this may be prevented. Similarly, entrainment does create dilution but this has not been demonstrated to be detrimental.

VI. CONCLUSIONS

HFV has been demonstrated to provide effective gas exchange during various types of surgical procedures over a wide range of frequencies. Selection for mechanical ventilatory support is based upon multiple factors, including the physical status of the patient, requirements of the clinical situation, the capability for providing appropriate oxygenation and ventilation, and potential physiologic advantages. Because HFV produces significantly lower peak airway pressures than CMV, it might prevent cardiac compromise and barotrauma. In addition, in cases allowing the insertion of a small catheter into the trachea, rather than a larger endotracheal tube, HFV may be superior. In surgical situations where tissue movement should be minimized, such as pediatric thoracic and microneurosurgery, HFJV may prove to be beneficial.

Even with these potential advantages, HFV — particularly HFJV — is intimately related to the characteristics of the patient's respiratory system. Changes in patient status may alter gas exchange; hence, close monitoring of arterial blood gas tensions and airway pressure is essential.

REFERENCES

1. Quan, S. F., Calkins, J. M., Waterson, C. K., and Otto, C. W., High frequency ventilation — current Concepts, *Ariz. Med.*, 40, 319, 1983.
2. Quan, S. F. and Calkins, J. M., High frequency ventilation — promising new method of ventilation, *Heart Lung*, 12, 152, 1983.
3. Sjostrand, U., Review of the physiological rationale for the development of high frequency positive pressure ventilation — HFPPV, *Acta Anaesth. Scand.*, Suppl. 64, 7, 1977.
4. Sjostrand, U., High frequency positive pressure ventilation (HFPPV): a review, *Crit. Care Med.*, 8, 345, 1980.
5. Carlon, G. C., Miodownik, S., Ray, C., Jr., et al., Technical aspects and clinical implications of high frequency jet ventilation with a solenoid valve, *Crit. Care Med.*, 9, 47, 1981.
6. Calkins, J. M., Waterson, C. K., Hameroff, S. R., Harris, T. R., and Jones, J. F., A simple flueric high frequency jet ventilator, *Anesth. Analg.*, 61, 138, 1982.
7. Klain, M. and Smith, R. B., High frequency percutaneous transtracheal jet ventilation, *Crit. Care Med.*, 5, 280, 1977.
8. Slutsky, A. S., Kamm, R. D., and Drazen, J. M., A review of experimental and theoretical studies of high frequency ventilation, in *Perspectives in High Frequency Ventilation*, Scheck, P. A., Sjostrand, U. H., and Smith, R. B., Eds., Martinus Nijhoff, Boston, 1983, 59.
9. Butler, W. J., Bohn, D. J., Bryan, A. C., et al., Ventilation by high frequency oscillation in humans, *Anesth. Analg.*, 59, 577, 1980.
10. Hameroff, S. R., Calkins, J. M., Waterson, C. K., et al., High frequency alternating lung ventilation, *Anesthesiology*, 54, 238, 1981.
11. Calkins, J. M. and Waterson, C. K., Clinical factors influencing the selection of HFJV, *Crit. Care Med.*, 12(9), 806, 1984.
12. Quan, S. F., Militzer, H. W., Calkins, J. M., and Waterson, C. K., High frequency ventilation applications in the OR, *AORN J.*, 38, 991, 1983.
13. Crawford, M. R. and Rehder, K., High frequency small volume ventilation (HFV) in anesthetized man, *Anesthesiology*, Suppl. 59, A503, 1983.
14. Calkins, J. M., Waterson, C. K., Hameroff, S. R., and Kanel, J., Jet pulse characteristics for high frequency jet ventilation in dogs, *Anesth. Analg.*, 61, 293, 1982.
15. Calkins, J. M., High frequency jet ventilation, in *Experimental Evaluation in High Frequency Ventilation*, Carlon, G. C., Eds., Marcel Dekker, New York, accepted for publication.
16. Pinchak, A. C., Hogen, J. F., Hancock, D. E., and Kovijanic, C., Beat frequencies in high frequency positive pressure ventilation, *Crit. Care Med.*, 12(9), 729, 1984.
17. Klain, M., Norolin, N., and Keszler, H., Microciliary transport with and without humidification in high frequency ventilation, *Anesthesiology*, 57, A86, 1982.
18. Smith, R. B., Schaer, W. B., and Pfaeffle, H., Percutaneous transtracheal ventilation for anaesthesia and resuscitation: a review and report of complications, *Can. Anaesth. Soc. J.*, 22, 607, 1975.
19. Klain, M., Keszler, H., and Stool, S., Transtracheal high frequency jet ventilation prevents aspiration, *Crit. Care Med.*, 11, 170, 1983.
20. Klain, M., Keszler, H., and Brader, E., High frequency jet ventilation in CPR, *Crit. Care Med.*, 9, 421, 1981.
21. Szele, G., Keenan, R. L., Does percutaneous transtracheal high frequency ventilation prevent aspiration? A word of caution, *Crit. Care Med.*, 9, 163, 1981.
22. Calkins, G. C., Pierri, M. K., Ray, C., and Kreton, V., Hemodynamic and respiratory variables with high frequency jet ventilation (HFJV) synchronized with heart rate, *Crit. Care Med.*, 9, 163, 1981.
23. Otto, C. W., Quan, S. F., Conahan, T. J., Calkins, J. M., Waterson, C. W., and Hameroff, S. R., Hemodynamic effects of high frequency jet ventilation, *Anesth. Analg.*, 62, 298, 1983.
24. Butler, W. J., Bohn, D. J., Bryan, A. C., and Froese, A. B., Ventilation by high frequency oscillation in humans, *Anesth. Analg.*, 59, 55, 1980.

25. Schuster, D. P., Snyder, J. V., Klain, M., and Grenvik, A., The use of high frequency jet ventilation during respiratory failure, *Crit. Care Med.*, 9, 162, 1981.
26. Dedhia, H. V., Hemodynamic effect of high frequency ventilation in open heart surgery patients, *Crit. Care Med.*, 9, 158, 1981.
27. Carlon, G. C., Pierri, M. K., Ray, C., and Kretan, V., Hemodynamic and respiratory variables with high frequency jet ventilation (HFJV) synchronized with heart rate, *Crit. Care Med.*, 9, 163, 1983.
28. Hoff, B. H., Robotham, J. L., Smith, R. B., Cherry, D., and Bunegin, L., Effects of high frequency ventilation (300 to 2400/min) on cardiovascular function and gas exchange in dogs, *Anesth. Analg.*, 60, 256, 1981.
29. Eriksson, I. A., Hoven, A., Sedin, G., and Sjostrand, V., The influence of the ventilatory pattern on ventilation, circulation, and oxygen transport during continuous positive pressure ventilation: an experimental study, *Acta Anaesth. Scand.*, Suppl. 64, 149, 1977.
30. Szele, G. and Shahvari, M. B. G., Comparison of cardiovascular effects of high frequency ventilation and intermittent positive pressure ventilation in hemorrhagic shock, *Crit. Care Med.*, 9, 161, 1981.
31. Carlon, G. C., Pierri, M. K., Ray, C., and Kreton, V., Hemodynamic and respiratory variables with high frequency jet ventilation (HFJV) synchronized with heart rate, *Crit. Care Med.*, 9, 163, 1981.
32. Calkins, J. M., Cork, R. C., and Militizer, H. W., Effect of high frequency ventilation on left ventricular function as measured by esophageal echocardiography, *Anesth. Suppl.*, 6(3A), 72, 1984.
33. Chiranda, M., Rubini, A., Fiore, G., Giron, G., and Carlon, G. C., Hemodynamic effects of continuous positive-pressure ventilation and high frequency jet ventilation with positive end-expiratory pressure in normal dogs, *Crit. Care Med.*, 12(9), 750, 1984.
34. Tabatabai, M. and Javadi, P., Comparison of hemodynamics with HFJV and IPPV during abdominal aortic operation, *Anesthesiology*, Suppl. 61, A67, 1984.
35. Todd, M. M., Toutant, S. M., and Shapiro, H. M., The effects of high frequency positive pressure ventilation on ICP and brain surface movement in cars, *Anesthesiology*, 54, 496, 1981.
36. Lobo, D. P., Brauer, F. S., Ciobanu, M., Hill, W., and Klein, O., High frequency jet ventilation in superficial temporal artery to middle cerebral artery, *Anesthesiology*, Suppl. 61, A319, 1984.
37. Grasberger, R. C., Spatz, E. L., Mortara, R. W., Ordia, J. I., and Yeston, N. S., Effect of high frequency ventilation vs conventional mechanical ventilation of ICP in head-injured dogs, *J. Neurosurg.*, 60, 1214, 1984.
38. Toutant, S. M., Todd, M. M., and Drummond, J. C., Cerebral blood flow during high frequency ventilation in cats, *Crit. Care Med.*, 11, 712, 1983.
39. Babinski, M. F., Albin, M., and Smith, R. B., Effect of high frequency ventilation in ICP, *Crit. Care Med.*, 9, 159, 1981.
40. Hoff, B. F., Benedetto, A. R., Nusynowitz, L., Wilson, E. A., and Smith, R. B., Rapid infusion air embolism: effects of IPPV and high frequency ventilation (HFJV), *Anesthesiology*, 57, A85, 1982.
41. Marquez, J., Klain, M., and Romabo, B., Renal and cardiovascular effects between CPAP and HFJV with PEEP, *Anesthesiology*, 55, A68, 1981.
42. Jonzon, A., High frequency positive pressure ventilation by endotracheal insufflation, *Acta Anaesth. Scand.*, Suppl. 43, 1, 1971.
43. Marquez, J., Guntupalli, K., Sladen, A., and Klain, M., Renal function and renin secretion during HFJV at varying levels of airway pressure, *Crit. Care Med.*, 11, 930, 1983.
44. Marquez, J., Fine, J., Klain, M., Bennett, R., and Freeman, J., Clinical applications of high frequency jet ventilation in the operating room, *Anesthesiology*, 57, A464, 1982.
45. Eriksson, I. A. and Sjostrand, U. H., HFPPV during bronchoscopy and laryngoscopy, in *High Frequency Ventilation*, Smith, R. B. and Sjostrand, U. H., Eds., Little, Brown, Boston, 1983, 63.
46. Smith, R. B. and Babinski, M. J., Clinical high frequency jet ventilation, in *High Frequency Ventilation*, Smith, R. B. and Sjostrand, U. H., Eds., Little, Brown, Boston, 1983, 89.
47. Versiechelen, L., Rolly, G., and Vermeersch, H., High frequency insufflation technique during endolaryngeal microsurgery, *in Perspectives in High Frequency Ventilation*, Scheck, P. A., Sjostrand, U. H., and Smith, R. B., Eds., Martinus Nijhoff, Boston, 1983, 188.
48. Scheck, P. A., Mallios, C., and Knegt, P., High frequency ventilation for laser surgery of the larynx, in *Perspectives in High Frequency Ventilation*, Scheck, P. A., Sjostrand, U. H., and Smith, R. B., Eds., Martinus Nijoff, Boston, 1984, 204.
49. Hirlinger, W. K., Deller, A., Sigg, O., Dick, W., and Mehrkens, H., High frequency jet ventilation via a vasotracheal tube for surgery of the larynx and trachea, in *Perspectives in High Frequency Ventilation*, Sheck, P. A., Sjostrand, U. H., and Smith, R. B., Eds., Martinus Nijhoff, Boston, 1984, 212.
50. Scheck, P. A. and Mallios, C., Peroral endoscopies using intravenous anesthesia and high frequency ventilation, *Crit. Care Med.*, 12(9), 803, 1984.
51. Borg, U., Eriksson, I., and Sjostrand, U., High frequency positive pressure ventilation (HFPPV): a review based upon its use during bronchoscopy and for laryngoscopy and microlaryngeal surgery under general anesthesia, *Anesth. Analg.*, 59, 594, 1980.

52. Sanders, R. D., Two ventilating attachments for bronchoscopes, *Del. Med. J.*, 39, 170, 1967.
53. Cole, W. H. J., Choice of anaesthetic technique for microsurgery of the larynx, *Anaesth. Intensive Care*, 3, 62, 1975.
54. Spoerel, W. E. and Grant, P. A., Ventilation during bronchoscopy, *Can. Anaesth. Soc.*, 18, 178, 1971.
55. Klain, M., Gas exchange in high frequency ventilation: an experimental study, in *Perspectives in High Frequency Ventilation*, Scheck, P. A., Sjostrand, U. J., and Smith, R. B., Eds., Martinus Nijhoff, Boston, 1983, 158.
56. Smith, R. B., Cutaia, F., Hoff, B. H., Babinski, M., and Geliveau, J., Long term transtracheal high frequency ventilation in dogs, *Crit. Care Med.*, 9, 311, 1981.
57. Hoff, B. H., Smith, R. B., and Bunegin, L., High frequency ventilation in dogs with open chests, *Crit. Care Med.*, 10, 517, 1982.
58. Carlon, G. C., Griffin, J., Ray, C., Groeger, J. S., and Patrick, K., High frequency jet ventilation in experimental airway disruptions, *Crit. Care Med.*, 11, 353, 1983.
59. El-Baz, N., El-Ganzouri, A., and Ivankovich, A., One-lung high frequency ventilation for intrathoracic surgery, in *Perspectives in High Frequency Ventilation*, Scheck, P. A., Sjostrand, U. A., and Smith, R. B., Eds., Martinus Nijhoff, Boston, 1983, 216.
60. El-Baz, N., El-Ganzouri, A., and Ivankovich, A., High frequency positive pressure ventilation for major surgery, in *Perspectives in High Frequency Ventilation*, Scheck, P. A., Sjostrand, U. A., and Smith, R. B., Eds., Martinus Nijhoff, Boston, 1983, 216.
61. Moulaert, P. and Rolly, G., High frequency jet ventilation for pulmonary resection, in *Perspectives in High Frequency Ventilation*, Scheck, P. A., Sjostrand, U. A., and Smith, R. B., Eds., Martinus Nijhoff, Boston, 1983, 227.
62. Mutz, N., Baum, M., Benzer, H., Holler, W., Mortiz, E., and Pauser, G., Intraoperative application of high frequency ventilation, *Crit. Care Med.*, 12(9), 800, 1984.
63. Lee, K., Abramsan, S., and Naik, N., Jet ventilation of one lung for laser resection of bronchial tumor, *Anesth. Analg.*, 63, 957, 1984.
64. Seki, S., Goto, K., Kondo, T., Fukushima, Y., Komishi, H., and Kosaka, F., Gas exchange and facilitation of high frequency ventilation in intrathoracic surgery, *Annals. Thorac. Surg.*, 37(6), 491, 1984.
65. Crawford, M. R. and Rehder, K., High frequency small volume ventilation (HFV) in thoracic surgery, *Anesthesiology*, Suppl., 61(3A), A507, 1984.
66. El-Baz, N., Jensik, R., Faber, L. P., and Faro, R. S., One-lung high frequency ventilation for tracheoplasty and bronchoplasty: a new technique, *Soc. Thorac. Surg.*, 34(5), 564, 1982.
67. El-Baz, N., Holinger, L., El-Ganzoni, A., Gottschalk, W., and Ivankovich, A. D., High frequency positive pressure ventilation for tracheal reconstruction supported by tracheal T-tube, *Anesth. Analg.*, 61(9), 796, 1982.
68. Smith, R. B., Hoff, B. H., Rosen, L., Wilson, E., and Swatzman, S., High frequency ventilation during pulmonary lobectomy: three cases, *Resp. Care*, 26(5), 437, 1981.
69. Prust, R. S. and Calkins, J. M., Considerations for managing the airway in the ENT patient, in *Contemporary Anesthesia Practice*, Vol. 9, Brown, B. R., Ed., in Press, chap. 9.
70. Ruder, C. B., et al., Anesthesia for carbon dioxide laser microsurgery of the larynx, *Otolaryng. Head Neck Surg.*, 89, 732, 1981.
71. Carden, E. and Ferguson, G. C., A new technique for microlaryngeal surgery in infants, *Laryngoscope*, 83, 691, 1973.
72. Carden, E., et al., A comparison of venture and side arm ventilation in anaesthesia for bronchoscopy, *Can. Anaesth. Soc. J.*, 20, 569, 1973.
73. Chaussy, C., Schuller, J., Schmiedt, E., Brandl, H., Jocham, D., and Liedl, B., Extracoporeal shockwave lithotripsy (ESWL) for treatment of urolithiasis, *Urology*, 23, 59, 1984.
74. Schulte am Esch, J., Kochs, E., and Meyer, W. H., Improved Efficiency of extracorporeal shock wave lithotripsy during high frequency jet ventilation, *Anesthesiol.*, Suppl. 63, A177, 1985.
75. Carlson, C. A., Boysen, P. G., Banner, M. J., and Gravenstein, J. S., Conventional versus high frequency jet ventilation for extracorporeal shock wave lithotripsy, *Anesthesiol.*, Suppl., 63, A530, 1985.

Chapter 11

COMPLICATIONS AND PATHOLOGY RELATED TO HIGH FREQUENCY VENTILATION

Robert A deLemos, Donald M. Mull, Jr., and Jacqueline J. Coalson

TABLE OF CONTENTS

I. INTRODUCTION

The term HFV refers to a groups of ventilatory techniques which share in common the use of rapid rates and small tidal volumes. In the lower frequency ranges (1 to 2 Hz, 60 to 120 cpm) neither gas exchange physiology nor the required technology are markedly different from that of conventional positive pressure ventilation. At the higher frequencies specially designed oscillators or flow interruptors must be designed and the altered pulmonary and nonpulmonary physiology leads to a variety of unique findings.[1-3]

The various techniques of HFV have generated considerable interest among clinicians of various disciplines. As they strive to find clinical applications for these innovative approaches to mechanical ventilation, investigators have usually emphasized the theoretic advantages and downplayed potential hazards. Most animal experiments have been short term, and human studies often are incapable of detecting subtle complications. Since in most instances conventional ventilation has been proven to be safe and effective, careful assessment of the risk to benefit ratio must be made before widespread use of HFV can be advocated.

Specially designed ventilators and ventilator circuits are required to safely use any of the HFV techniques. Attempts to modify either the circuit or the ventilator should be accompanied by adequate in vitro testing of the redesigned system before it is used in humans. Seemingly insignificant changes such as the relocation of the jet catheter during HFV or the placement of a different connector or water trap in a HFOV circle may dramatically alter the characteristics of an HFV ventilator.[4-7]

Conventional positive pressure ventilators are designed to function optimally in the physiologic range of ventilatory frequency. System compliance is relatively insignificant because tidal volume is presumed to be large in proportion; likewise, the timing systems and responsiveness of the exhalation valves are designed for relatively low frequencies. Attempts to convert commercially available positive pressure ventilators to "high frequency" by altering the cycling mechanism usually results in poor response or clinical disaster. Hypoventilation, dynamic increase in functional residual capacity, pulmonary hypertension, and acute right heart failure are among the complications of this inappropriate maneuver.[8-11]

One major difference between HFV of any type and conventional positive pressure ventilation is related to the rapid frequency and the requirement for instantaneous response in situations where the system develops excessive pressure. Equipment failures such as occlusion of the exhalation limb of an oscillator circle or mucous impaction in the endotracheal tube during jet ventilation may result in rapid overpressurization of the system with pulmonary overdistension and rupture. Acute cor pulmonale and cardiac arrest may ensue.[12,13] To avoid this, all HFV must be monitored with a high pressure sensor and a servo-controlled device which immediately opens the patient circle to ambient gas at atmospheric pressure. Low pressure, bias flow, power loss, and inspiratory duration alarms are also desirable.

Even when open patient circles are used during HFV, delivered tidal volumes along with lung and ventilator time constants are important in the determination of the effective functional residual capacity. Rouby, Franz and others have reported a dynamic increase in FRC during jet ventilation, particularly, when jet volume is large and the inspiratory duration is relatively long.[14,15] Although less common, an inadvertent increase in FRC has also been seen during HFOV under some conditions. Although there may be some mechanical advantage of the "active" exhalation phase during HFO, in general the prinicple that there must be sufficient time for gas egress applies to all ventilators and frequencies. With inadequate time for exhalation there will be an inapparent increase in FRC with an increased risk of baroinjury, hypoventilation, and acute cor pulmonale. Under these circumstances measurement of proximal MAP will not accurately reflect either alveolar mean pressure or lung volume.[16-21] Direct measurement or monitoring of mean lung volume will provide adequate safeguards particularly in infants, or patients with relatively compliant lungs.

Finally, a unique problem can arise during oscillatory ventilation if the combination of a low MAP and a large oscillatory volume results in subambient pressures at the oropharynx. When this occurs in patients with diffuse alveolar disease (DAD), it results in rapid clinical deterioration from alveolar collapse.[95]

II. CARDIOVASCULAR COMPLICATIONS

Much of the early enthusiasm for the use of HFV in intra- and postoperative cardiac surgery stemmed from observations that many of the adverse effects of PPV (positive pressure ventilation) on cardiac output were modified or eliminated during HFV.[22,23] These favorable effects are present only if lung volumes remain normal. In situations where alveolar overdistension occurs as a consequence of inadvertent gas trapping from HFV there may be a dramatic increase in the mechanical component of pulmonary vascular resistance with an increase in pulmonary artery pressure and right heart strain. Hoff et al.[24] has described an interaction between left ventricular stroke output and lung inflation during both spontaneous and conventional positive pressure breathing. This enhancement of left ventricular function is absent during HFV, but its absence has no apparent adverse effect on the normal heart.[25-28] When HFOV is used in the treatment of DAD, one strategy is to use a high MAP to minimize intrapulmonary shunting.[29] In this situation the limiting factor is cardiac output and many patients will not tolerate this maneuver. Unfortunately there are little data comparing HFV to conventional ventilation in patients with pre-existing myocardial dysfunction. Until more is available the specific effect of HFV on cardiac function will have to be measured directly.

Under certain circumstances the absence of cyclical ventilatory effects on pulmonary vascular resistance may have a negative impact. Infants and children with intracardiac and extracardiac left-to-right shunts often benefit from PPV. The increased pulmonary vascular resistance during lung inflation decreases the magnitude of the shunt.[30] When HFOV and HFFI (high frequency flow interruptor) are used in the premature baboon with hyaline membrane disease, clinical problems associated with ductal left-to-right shunt are more prevalent.[31] Flow doppler studies in animals and humans reveal an absence of retrograde flow during ventilator inspiration with PPV but persistence throughout the ventilatory cycle during HFV.[32] Thus PPV appears to be more effective in controlling the magnitude of a left-to-right shunt in the newborn and ductal ligation may be necessary if HFV is to be used in the treatment of infants with hyaline membrane disease (HMD). Finally, the efficacy of HFV in the ventilator management of pulmonary edema has not been defined. The high, near constant alveolar pressures required to manage pulmonary edema with HFV may themselves decrease venous return and cardiac output.

We have observed hepatic and cerebral venous engorgement in animals treated with HPOV, leading to the possibility that the absence of fluctuating extrapleural pressures decreases venous return.

III. PULMONARY COMPLICATIONS

It was originally assumed that during HFV, distal airway pressures would be significantly lower than proximal pressures with HFV offering a means of reducing the incidence of pulmonary barotrauma.[33-35] Models based on the assumption that alveolar compliance was normal, predicted a reduced pressure amplitude in smaller airways during HFV.[36] However, high peak pressures have been measured in distal airways when distal exchange units are noncompliant or airways are obstructed. Mean alveolar pressures have also been found to be higher that proximal airway pressures.[16,37]

Although a comparison of HFJV and volume cycled ventilation showed less hyperinflation and no significant atelectasis with HFV,[38] visual observations by Carlon and co-workers showed that collapsed lung segments re-expanded and remained distended despite the low tidal volumes delivered with HFJV.[39,40] The relevance of these observations may account for some of the complications that have arisen in several reported studies described below.

The use of HFV in experimental animals with low compliance due to pulmonary immaturity and a lack of adequate surfactant has yielded interesting data.[41-44] An *appropriate* high frequency ventilatory strategy is capable of providing ventilatory support to premature baboons with hyaline membrane disease.[95] In a comparison of PPV/PEEP and HFV using both oscillation and the flow interruptor in the premature baboon with RDS for 2 hr periods, HFV resulted in better oxygenation at lower proximal airway pressures. However, attempts to carry these studies beyond 2 hr revealed that while PPV/PEEP animals did well, the HFV baboons, after 6 to 8 hr of excellent blood gases, developed hypoxemia, progressive hypercarbia, and severe diffuse atelectasis. When a left to right shunt through the ductus arteriosus was present, ductal flow was greater in the HFV animals.[42]

The interposition of an intermittent large inflation (sigh) stabilized the animals on HFV and ultimately resulted in good survival with this technique. However, the timing and volume of the sigh were found to be critical, and excessive volume or superimposition of the sigh before lung volume reached FRC resulted in airway disruption and pulmonary interstitial emphysema.[43] When a "controlled" sigh during HFV was compared with conventional ventilation in premature baboons with RDS, all animals in both groups survived. The animals on high frequency required less oxygen, were maintained at a lower MAP, and had more uniform saccular inflation at the end of the 24 hr experimental period.[42]

An extended 96 hr study again verified that HFV yielded better oxygenation at lower MAP when compared to conventional ventilation.[41] Also, the HFFI and HFO animals had higher a/AO_2 ratios than the PPV group, suggesting that the high frequency treated animals had saccular recruitment earlier than those treated with PPV. Comparing the two high frequency groups showed that the animals on the flow interruptor were better oxygenated at lower pressures that were the animals on the oscillator during the first 48 hr of the experiment. In spite of this lowered *proximal* MAP in the HFFI animals, a pathologic finding of a "junctional" hemorrhage was found more frequently in this group.[41] Its occurrence at the bronchiolar-saccular junction may be related to the tissue stress induced during the recruitment of poorly compliant alveoli since this area is known to be more susceptible to sheer forces.[45,46] The occurrence of these hemorrhages in the experimental group with the earliest clinical improvement may have been a result of rapid opening of airway units having increased surface tension.

These observations have been extended over longer periods in our laboratory. Although both HFFI and HPOV result in better oxygenation at lower proximal mean pressures than does PPV, lungs of animals treated with HFFI have pathologic evidence of barotrauma of a degree comparable to those treated with conventional ventilation. This probably was related to inadvertent air trapping at the frequency (10 Hz 600 cpm) and tidal volume used, but again emphasizes the importance of expiratory time constants in determining the strategy for a particular HFV device.

In another HFV study on nonhuman primates, Truog and co-workers examined the effects of 24 hr of HFOV on premature monkeys using a frequency of 10 to 20 Hz (600 to 1200 cpm) and an airway pressure of 10 cm H_2O or greater.[44] They found that high frequency oscillation yielded lower arterial PCO_2's at 6 and 12 hr study periods, but no differences were seen in arterial to inspired PO_2 ratios, or total lung phospholipids between the high frequency and conventionally ventilated groups.

Additional studies in experimental adult animals which were made surfactant deficient to determine whether HFV would augment or prevent the development of lung lesions are contradictory and confusing. Hamilton and co-workers used a surface active material (SAM) depleted adult rabbit model and showed that HFOV maintained excellent gas exchange when compared to animals treated with conventional ventilation.[47] In addition, the rabbits treated with high frequency show little pulmonary cellular damage when compared to the conventionally ventilated group. Using a comparable lung injury model in rabbits, Quan et al. studied animals treated with HFJV, conventional ventilation, and combined conventional and HFJV.[48] Their data showed no statistically significant differences among the three study groups with respect to survival, incidence of pneumothorax, or metabolic acidosis. Of special note, the pathologic findings in the three groups were comparable and included hyaline membranes, alveolar edema, and alveolar granulocytes. Whether these differences mean that there is less injury using oscillation in preference to jet ventilation has not been verified.

In the SAM-depleted adult lung models, oxygenation has been found to be better in the high frequency jet or oscillation-ventilated groups when compared to animals treated with conventional ventilation [47,48] with one exception.[49] Jibelian and Burkhard used repeated lavages to produce a surfactant deficient lung in mongrel dogs and showed, using HFPV and comparing it to conventional ventilation, that the high frequency stratagem was not effective in supporting gas exchange. They suggested that critical opening pressures were higher in the diseased lungs requiring delivery of higher airway pressures for efficient ventilation.

Other experimental studies using a different type of injury have suggested that HFV might be less effective in pathologic lungs than in normal lungs. Thompson et al. compared high frequency oscillation and conventional ventilation in the treatment of oleic acid induced lung injury in beagles and found high frequency oscillation to be less effective.[28] Gallagher and Banner also used an oleic acid lung injury in dogs and reported that HFJV resulted in decreased P_aO_2 and increased venous admixture at constant Paw and PEEP levels.[50] A third study by Schuster et al. compared high frequency to conventional ventilation in dogs with oleic acid induced pulmonary edema and found that PO_2 in high frequency treated animals was consistently lower than in conventionally ventilated controls.[51]

The differences in results in the two lung injury models are striking and not easily explained on a pathologic basis. The surfactant depleted lung would be expected to show diffuse alveolar injury where oleic acid yields a diffusely focal pulmonary edema. The most likely answer lies in differences in HFV strategy among the various experiments. When HFV is used in the management of diffuse alveolar damage, oxygenation is dependent on the mean lung volume. None of these studies attempted to control this variable and are therefore not comparable. Using HFV in the baboon with hyaline membrane disease, at an equivalent proximal MAP oxygenation is as good or better during HFV as compared to PPV.

The overall effect of HFV on the prevalence of pulmonary complications can only be tested in controlled experiments in human or appropriate animal models. The various strategic decisions which must be made in the use of any ventilatory approach will determine the relative risk or complications. For example, it is clear, as already stated, that high MAP will improve oxygenation during HFV. Airway disruption and cardiovascular compromise increase with increasing mean pressure. The risk:benefit ratio of each of the HFV stratagems and techniques will have to be closely evaluated before the real incidence of lung complications can be known.

There are studies which examine HFV at frequencies between 1 and 3 Hz in infants and adults. Eyal et al. treated 25 newborn infants with severe respiratory failure using HFPPV at 1.5 to 3.0 Hz.[5] The P_aO_2 increased and P_aCO_2 decreased in all infants within 1 hr, data which are comparable to those in some experimental nonhuman primate studies.[41,42] With this high frequency stratagem MAP were usually less than or equal to the pressures noted with conventional ventilation. The complications in this human study included pneumothorax in two patients and bronchopulmonary dysplasia (BPD) in one patient. Of the infants surviving (72%), none died of respiratory failure. In another clinical study, Bland and workers used rates between 1 and 1.8 Hz in 24 infants with severe hyaline membrane disease.[53] They noted that improvement was further enhanced by using manual ventilation at 3 Hz, a technique described by Ng in the successful management of bilateral interstitial emphysema,[54] (92% of the infants survived). Pulmonary complications included pneumothoraces in two patients, hemorrhage in three patients, postextubation lobar atelectasis in seven patients, and persistent respiratory distress in four patients.

Clinical studies designed to evaluate HFV as a ventilatory strategy in patients with adult respiratory distress syndrome (ARDS) have been inconclusive. There are no reliable indicators to predict which patients with respiratory failure will benefit from conventional or HFV. Carlon et al. recently re-examined this question and have offered an approach in the ventilatory management of patients in respiratory failure.[55] No unusual complications of HFV have surfaced in the ARDS population, although the problem of nonresponsiveness to HFV in certain patients has been noted.

The problem of air leaks developing during HFV is recognized, but is of no greater magnitude than that which occurs during conventional ventilation.[52] The use of the high gas flows in jet ventilation relies on an open system for gas egress, otherwise rapid and massive lung over-inflation can occur. This is clinically of great import when dealing with patients having upper airway obstruction. There are several reports that examine expiratory time constants and their relationship to the development of barotrauma.[56,57] Heicher and workers,[56] and Primhak[57] have indicated that a short inspiratory time is an essential factor in the prevention of barotrauma. As noted before, the timing and volume of any superimposed large volume breath (sigh) are critical, and excessive volume or superimposition of the sigh before lung volume reaches FRC can result in airway disruption and pulmonary interstitial emphysema (PIE).[43]

Tracheal injury has been recognized as a potential complication following any type of assisted ventilation. However, HFJV is felt to have an increased potential for erosive tracheal lesions due to the "jackhammer" effect of the dry high pressure jet stream of gas on the tracheal mucosa.[58,59] Oscillatory ventilation has revealed only focal tracheal epithelial ulceration and squamous metaplastic changes similar to those seen with conventional ventilation and probably related only to endotracheal intubation.[95] Humidification has proved to be of utmost importance especially with the use of the HFJV. Pokora reported on ten neonates with respiratory failure who received HFJV.[60] Of the six patients treated with HFJV for more than 20 hr three developed severe tracheal obstruction from thick tenacious secretions. These authors speculated that the observed tracheal damage was due to inadequately humidified gas rather than to jet induced trauma. Other workers have failed to demonstrate any significant tracheal damage in either animal or adult patients.[61,62] A study of Doyle and workers has compared the efficacy of four different humidification systems in dogs during a 24 hr study period using HFJV.[63] All animal groups which received some type of humidification showed no apparent change in epithelial or cilial histology in either the trachea or bronchi. The newborn appears to be unusually susceptible to injury during jet ventilation. Important factors in minimizing this risk appear to be adequate humidification, appropriate direction of the jet entry port, and avoidance of entrainment volume. To date, there are no long term animal or human studies verifying the safety of an optimally designed jet ventilator for newborn applications.

Mucus plugging has been described in a number of HFV studies. Whether it results from inadequate humidification of from disruption of normal mucociliary movement during HFV has not been established. There is conflicting evidence on the effect of HFV on mucociliary clearance. McEvoy and his co-workers compared IPPV and HFV on the clearance of a radiolabeled isotope delivered to the airways of dogs.[64] Their results indicated IPPV was more efficient in clearing the radiolabeled colloid; in fact, nearly all the isotope remained in the lung following 4 hr of HFV. Tracheal mucous clearance has also been shown to decrease during HFV when compared to spontaneous respiration and conventional ventilation.[65,66] Other investigators in test lung systems have observed outward movement of particles during HFOV. Regardless of the cause of the mucus plugging, its occurrence in patients receiving either high frequency jet or oscillatory ventilation has been noted by multiple investigators.[60] Mucus plugging during ventilatory support of neonates and its presence has been documented at postmortem not only as mucus within airways but also as mucus pools in peripheral air spaces, not related to any pneumonitic process.[95] Some infants with marked clinical abnormalities from diffuse plugging have been successfully managed with *N*-acetylcysteine while on HFV.

It is paradoxical that while HFV may lead to mucus plugging in some conditions, in several others where mucus plugs are a significant part of the primary disease process, improvement has been noted following HFV.[67] Patients with cystic fibrosis and chronic obstructive lung disease have shown improvement following treatment with HFPPV. Whether this improvement results from the vibratory effect of high frequency or is due to the potential of the HFV to deliver humidification and/or medications to the distal airways has not been established.

There have been few studies designed to examine alterations in surfactant during HFV. Aberrations in SAM have been described in states of hypo- and hyperventilation.[68-71] Large tidal volume inflations have been shown to lead to increased release of SAM from alveolar epithelial cells.[72-76] Truog et al. examined lung phospholipids in premature monkeys with HMD following 24 hr of HFOV or conventional ventilation and found no change in lung homogenate phospholipid, desaturated phosphatidycholine, or airway lavage phospholipid.[44] There was also no demonstrable difference in the percent of desaturated phosphatidycholine. In another study, Frantz examined lung or lavage surfactant active material in healthy adult cats following 6 hr of oscillatory or conventional ventilation and found no differences.[77] Mannino and co-workers have reported that the secretion of SAM from lamellar bodies into the alveolus and re-uptake of SAM from the alveolus is increased with HFOC.[78] Using the 100% oxygen-treated premature baboon model, animals ventilated with high frequency oscillation have increased quantities of lamellar inclusion bodies within the alveolar spaces when compared to conventional PPV or flow-interruptor ventilated groups.[95] Two mechanisms could be responsible; increased secretion secondary to the 100% oxygen injury, and/or enhanced release following the stimulation of the high frequency oscillations. With the data available there appears to be no functionally significant abnormality of surfactant related to the use of HFV. More detailed studies are needed to define more subtle changes in synthesis or turnover.

Lung weights, lung lymph flow, and the presence of pleural fluid have been examined by several investigators. Frantz and his co-workers examined healthy adult cats using HFOV and compared them to animals ventilated with conventional ventilation.[77] Their measurements showed no change in lung wet:dry weight ratios between the two groups. Truog and workers also found no difference in lung wet:dry weight ratios in high frequency or conventionally ventilated premature monkeys with hyaline membrane disease.[44] However, both study groups did have more liquid in their lungs when compared to animals without hyaline membrane disease. Raj and co-workers examined lung lymph fluid flow in healthy infant lambs in a 6 to 8 hr study period using HFV.[79] They showed a decrease in lung lymph flow during HFV, but the higher mean pulmonary arterial pressures evident in their HFV animals might have affected fluid movement in the interstitial compartment of the lung. Increased amounts of free pleural fluid were found by Rehder and associates who used HFOV for 24 to 36 hr in both healthy and sick dogs while dogs ventilated with IPPV showed no fluid.[80] In this same study, atelectasis was found in the lower lobes in 9 of 11 animals who received HFV, and in both lower lobes in two of the five dogs receiving conventional ventilation. It is not clear whether a sigh was used during HFV in these 36 hr studies.

IV. CNS COMPLICATIONS

To date, studies on the effects of HFV on intracranial pressure, cerebral blood flow and associated cardiac output have revealed no significant alterations.[81-83] However, at high frequencies HFOV results in almost constant pleural pressure, similar to that seen with high PEEP. PEEP can affect the distribution of systemic blood flow and may result in extra-thoracic venous engorgement and intracranial venous hypertension. The immature newborn may develop rupture of the periventricular plexus with hemorrhage if this occurs during HFOV. No clinical data are yet available but the theoretical risk is clearly present.

V. RENAL COMPLICATIONS

Renal function and renin secretion have been examined in patients receiving HFV at varying levels of airway pressure.[84] In patients receiving PEEP during HFJV, increased plasma renin level was noted and a decrease in stroke volume and cardiac indices were seen. Patients experienced decreased urinary flow, creatinine clearance and fractional excretion of sodium when compared to those who were treated with HFJV at zero and expiratory pressure.[84] PEEP is frequently associated with a reduced urine output and with sodium and water retention.[85] These changes have been thought to be caused by a release of antidiuretic hormone and a decrease in renal perfusion; however, some workers have shown that cardiac output and renal blood flow can be normal and have suggested that a third mechanism may be operative, an elevated airway pressure which would increase inferior vena cava and renal vein pressures. This in turn would cause redistribution of intrarenal blood flow and subsequently reduce urine and sodium excretion.

In the premature HMD baboon model, azotemia and oliguria are often seen, particularly in association with a persistent ductus arteriosus. By 96 hr with either HFOV, HFFI, or conventional ventilation, a consistent renal lesion is found consisting of varying sized hyaline droplets which completely fill the cytoplasm of the lower cortical tubular epithelial cells.[86]

VI. LIVER COMPLICATIONS

The development of severe fatty change and/or cytoplasmic vacuolization/edema in premature baboons ventilated with high frequency oscillation for a 96 hr study period was recently described.[87] Comparably severe lesions were not seen with the use of conventional or flow interruptor ventilators which allow an inflation-deflation pattern more consistent with normal ventilation. The cause(s) of these hepatic lesions probably relate to the PEEP-like effects elicited by high frequency oscillation.

Deterioration of hepatic function has been associated with increased airway pressures. Bushnell and his colleagues found that 30% of their patients receiving control conventional ventilation and 75% of those receiving PEEP had increased serum bilirubin values.[88] This was thought to be due to the downward displacement of the diaphragm followed by splanchnic hemodynamic disturbances were manifested as an increase in portal venous flow.[89-91]

Other investigators have found that a decrease in cardiac output can give rise to liver injury in human newborns. Infants with congenital heart disease, especially left-sided obstructive lesions, showed fatty change and hepatic cell necrosis.[92-94] It is known that the infant liver is more dependent upon systemic perfusion than portal flow, thus making it more susceptible to any decrease in cardiac output. The renal and hepatic dysfunction noted in some HFV studies may result from the above described circulatory changes.

VII. SUMMARY

Complete understanding of the potential complications of HFV are limited by a lack of carefully controlled long term experimental data. The clinical setting, where patients on ventilatory support often have complex multiple organ disease, is a difficult area in which to discover subtle consequences of any new technology. The best approach would be to test these new techniques in controlled long term studies using well designed animal models. Any problems detected could then be assessed in terms of risk benefit ratio in specific human clinical applications.

REFERENCES

1. Popovich, J. Jr., High-frequency ventilation, *Respir. Ther.*, 85, 3, 1983.
2. Sjostrand, U. H. and Eriksson, I. A., High rates and low volumes in mechanical ventilation — not just a matter of ventilatory frequency, *Anesth. Analg.*, 59(8), 567, 1980.
3. Ackerman, N. B. and deLemos, R. A., High frequency ventilation in, *Advances in Pediatrics* Vol. 31, Barness, L. A., Ed., Year Book, Chicago, 1984, 259.
4. Keszler, H. and Klain, M., Importance of jet orifice in high frequency jet ventilation, *Crit. Care Med.*, 10, 234, 1982.
5. Baum, M., Benzer, H., Geyer, A., et al., Gas exchange and flow properties during high frequency jet ventilation, *Crit. Care Med.*, 9, 159, 1981.
6. Lehnert, B. F., Overdorser, G., and Slutsky, A. S., Constant flow ventilation of apneic dogs, *J. Appl. Physiol.*, 53, 483, 1982.
7. Carlon, G. C., Miodownik, S., Ray, C. J., et al., Technical aspects and clinical implications of hgh frequency jet ventilation with a solenoid valve, *Crit. Care Med.*, 9, 47, 1981.
8. Boros, S. J. and Campbell, K., A comparison of the effects of high-frequency low tidal volume and low-frequency high tidal volume mechanical ventilation, *J. Pediatr.*, 97, 1980.
9. Boros, S. J., Mammel, M. D., Hagen, E., et. al., Infant ventilator performance: effects of altering frequency, peak inspiratory pressure, I:E ratio and PEEP, *Pediatr. Res.*, 17, 372A, 1983.
10. Brady, J., Deming, D. D., and McCann, E. M., Is rapid ventilation better?, *Clin. Res.*, 31, 133A, 1983.
11. Fontan, J. P., Heldt, G. P., Willis, M. W., et. al., Changes in functional residual capacity and inadvertent end expiratory pressure in rabbits ventilated at rapid rates, *Pediatr. Res.*, 17, 375A, 1983.
12. Miodownik, S., Ray, C., Jr., Carlon, G. C., et. al., High-frequency jet ventilation: technical implications, *Crit. Care Med.*, 12(9), 718, 1984.
13. Calkins, J. M. and Waterson, C. K., Clinical factors influencing the selection of high-frequency jet ventilators, *Crit. Care Med.*, 12(9), 806, 1984.

14. Rouby, J. J., Fusciardi, J., et. al., High frequency jet ventilation in post operative respiratory failure, *Anesthesiology,* 59, 281, 1983.
15. Franz, I. and Close, R., Elevated lung volume and alveolar pressure during jet ventilation of rabbits, *Am. Rev. Respir. Dis.,* 131, 134, 1985.
16. Ackerman, N. B. Jr., Null, D. M. Jr., et. al., Airway pressures during high frequency ventilation, *Pediatr. Res.,* 16, 344A, 1982.
17. Allen, J. L., Keefe, D. H., Fredberg, J. J., et. al., Alveolar pressures and pulmonary impedence during high frequency ventilation in excised rabbit lungs, *Pediatr. Res.,* 17, 370A, 1982.
18. Fletcher, P. R. and Epstein, R. A., Measurement of alveolar pressures during HFV, *Anesthesiology,* 55, 358A, 1981.
19. Beamer, W. C., Prouch, D. S., Rayster, R. L., et. al., High-frequency jet ventilation produces Auto-PEEP, *Crit. Care Med.,* 12(9), 734, 1984.
20. Groeger, J. S., Carlon, G. C., Howland, W. S., et. al., Experimental evaluation of high-frequency jet ventilation, *Crit. Care Med.,* 12(9), 734, 1984.
21. Carlon, G. C., Ray, C. Jr., Miodownik, S., et. al., Physiologic implications of high frequency jet ventilation techniques, *Crit. Care Med.,* 11, 508, 1983.
22. Oberg, P. A. and Sjostrand, U. H., Studies of blood pressure regulation III. Dynamics of arterial blood pressure on carotid-sinus nerve stimulation, *Acta Physiol. Scand.,* 81, 96.
23. Jonzon, A., Oberg, A., et. al., High-frequency positive-pressure ventilation by endotracheal insufflation, *Acta Anesth. Scand.,* Suppl. 43.
24. Hoff, B. H., Robotham, J. L., Smith, R. B., et. al., Effect of high frequency ventilation (300—2400/min) on cardiovascular function and gas exchange in dogs, *Am. Rev. Respir. Dis.,* 123, 108, 1981.
25. Chiaranda, M., Rubini, A., and Fiore, G., Hemodynamic effects of continuous positive-pressure ventilation and high frequency jet ventilation with positive end-expiratory pressure in normal dogs, *Crit. Care Med.,* 12(19), 750, 1984.
26. Klain, M. and Smith, R. B., High frequency percutaneous transtracheal jet ventilation, *Crit. Care Med.,* 5, 280, 1977.
27. Sjostrand, U. H. and Eriksson, E. A., High rates and low volumes in mechanical ventilation not just a matter of ventilatory frequency, *Anesth. Analg.,* 59, 567, 1980.
28. Thompson, W. K., Marchak, B. E., et. al., High-frequency oscillation compared with standard ventilation in pulmonary injury model, *J. Appl. Physiol.,* 52(3), 543, 1982.
29. Froese, A., Personal communication.
30. Roos, A., Thomas, L. J., Nagel, E. L., et. al., Pulmonary vascular resistance as determined by lung inflation and vascular pressures, *J. Appl. Physiol.,* 16, 77, 1961.
31. Ackerman, N. B. Jr., Kuehl, T. J., et. al., Cardiovascular interactions with high frequency ventilation: preliminary observations in premature baboons with hyaline membrane disease, *Crit. Care Med.,* 12, 338, 1984.
32. Yoder, B. A., Ackerman, N. B., Jr., et. al., The effect of mechanical ventilation on left to right ductal shunting in immature baboons, *Crit. Care Med.,* 12, 376, 1984.
33. Bohn, D. J., Miyasaka, K., Marchak, B. E., Thompson, W. K., Froese, A. B., and Bryan, A. C., Ventilation by high-frequency oscillation, *J. Appl. Physiol.,* 48, 710, 1980.
34. Frantz, D. D., III, Werthammer, J., and Stark, A. R., High-frequency ventilation in premature infants with lungs diseases: adequate gas exchange at low tracheal pressure, *Pediatrics,* 71, 483, 1983.
35. Slutsky, A. S., Drazen, J. M., Ingram, R. H., Jr., Kamm, R. D., Shapiro, A. H., Fredberg, J. J., Loring, S. H., and Lehr, J., Effective pulmonary ventilation with small-volume oscillations at high frequency, *Science,* 209, 609, 1980.
36. Scherer, P. W. and Haselton, F. R., Convective exchange and oscillatory flow through bronchial-tree models, *J. Appl. Physiol.,* 53, 1023, 1982.
37. Allen, J. L., Keefe, D. H., Fredberg, J. J., Glass, G. M., and Frantz, I. D., Alveolar pressure and pulmonary impedance during high frequency oscillation in excised rabbit lungs, *Pediatr. Res.,* 17, 307a, 1983.
38. Slutsky, A. S., Kamm, R. D., and Drazen, J. M., High frequency oscillatory ventilation using tidal volumes smaller than the anatomical dead space, in *High Frequency Ventilation,* Smith, R. B. and Sjostrand, U. H., Eds., Little, Brown, Boston, 1983.
39. Turnbull, A. D., Carlon, G. C., Howland, W. S., and Beattie, E. J., Jr., High-frequency jet ventilation in major airway or pulmonary disruption, *Ann. Thorac. Surg.,* 32, 468, 1981.
40. Carlon, G. C., Griffin, J., Ray, C., Groeger, J., and Patrick, K., High frequency jet ventilation in experimental airway disruption, *Crit. Care Med.,* 11, 353, 1983.
41. Bell, R. E., Kuehl, T. J., Coalson, J. J., Escobedo, M. B., Yoder, B. A., Minnick, L. C., Stoddard, R., Meredith, K., Hilliard, J. L., Smith, F., Cipriani, C., Null, D. M., Robotham, J. L., and deLemos, R. A., High frequency ventilation compared to conventional positive-pressure ventilation in the treatment of hyaline membrane disease in primates, *Crit. Care Med.,* 12, 764, 1984.

42. Kuehl, T. J., Coalson, J. J., Ackerman, N. B., Escobedo, M. B., Bell, R., Yoder, B., Minnick, L., Stoddard, R., Meredith, K., Hilliard, J. L., Smith, F., Cipriani, C., Null, D. M., Robotham, J. L., and deLemos, R., High frequency ventilation in the treatment of hyaline membrane disease: the use of a baboon model to determine an acceptable ventilatory strategy, *Pediatrics,* in press.
43. Ackerman, N. B., Coalson, J. J., Kuehl, T. J., Stoddard, R., Minnick, L., Escobedo, M. B., Null, D. M., Robotham, J. L., and deLemos, R. A., Pulmonary interstitial emphysema in the premature baboon with hyaline membrane disease, *Crit. Care Med.,* 12, 512, 1984.
44. Truog, W. E., Standaert, T. A., Murphy, J. H., Woodrum, D. E., and Hodson, W. A., Effects of prolonged high-frequency oscillatory ventilation in premature primates with experimental hyaline membrane disease, *Am. Rev. Respir. Dis.,* 130, 76, 1984.
45. Lai-Fook, S. J. and Kallock, M. J., Bronchial-arterial interdependence in isolated dog lung, *J. Appl. Physiol.,* 52, 1000, 1982.
46. Mead, J., Takishima, T., and Leith, D., Stress distribution in lungs: a model of pulmonary elasticity, *J. Appl. Physiol.,* 28, 596, 1970.
47. Hamilton, P. P., Onayemi, A., Smyth, J. A., Gillan, J. E., Cutz, E., Froese, A. B., and Bryan, A. C., Comparison of conventional and high-frequency ventilation: oxygenation and lung pathology, *J. Appl. Physiol.,* 55, 131, 1983.
48. Quan, S. F., Militzer, H. W., Calkins, J. M., Sobonya, R. E., Waterson, C. K., Otto, C. W., and Conahan, T. J., Comparison of high-frequency jet ventilation with conventional mechanical ventilation in saline-lavaged rabbits, *Crit. Care Med.,* 12, 759, 1984.
49. Jibelian, G. and Burkkhard, L., Gas exchange during conventional and high frequency pulse ventilation in the surfactant-deficient lung: influence of positive end-expiratory pressure, *Crit. Care Med.,* 12, 769, 1984.
50. Gallagher, T. J. and Banner, M. J., High frequency positive pressure ventilation for oleic acid induced lung injury, *Crit. Care Med.,* 8, 232a, 1980.
51. Schuster, D. P., Snyder, J. V., and Klain, M., Comparison of venous admixture during high-frequency ventilation and conventional ventilation in oleic acid-induced pulmonary edema in dogs, *Anesth. Analg.,* 61, 735, 1982.
52. Eyal, F. G., Arad, I. D., Godder, K., and Robinson, M. J., High-frequency positive-pressure ventilation in neonates, *Crit. Care Med.,* 12, 793, 1984.
53. Bland, R. D., Kim, M. H., Light, M. J., and Woodson, J. L., High frequency mechanical ventilation in severe hyaline membrane disease, *Crit. Care Med.,* 8, 275, 1980.
54. Ng, K. P. K. and Easa, D., Management of interstitial emphysema by high frequency low positive-pressure hand ventilation in the neonate, *J. Pediatr.,* 95, 117, 1979.
55. Carlon, G. C., Howland, W. S., Groeger, J. S., Ray, C., and Miodownik, S., Role of high-frequency jet ventilation in the management of respiratory failure, *Crit. Care Med.,* 12, 777, 1984.
56. Heicher, D. A., Kasting, D. S., and Harrod, Jr., Prospective clinical comparison of two methods of mechanical ventilation of neonates: rapid rate and short inspiratory time versus slow rate and long inspiratory time, *J. Pediatr.,* 98, 957, 1981.
57. Primhak, R. A., Factors associated with pulmonary air leak in premature infants receiving mechanical ventilation, *J. Pediatr.,* 102, 764, 1983.
58. Nordin, U. L. F., Klain, M., and Kesvler, H., Electron microscopic studies of tracheal mucosa after high frequency jet ventilation, *Crit. Care Med.,* 10, 211, 1982.
59. Ophoven, J. P., Mammel, M. C., Gordon, M. J., and Boros, S. J., Tracheobronchial histopathology associated with high-frequency jet ventilation, *Crit. Care Med.,* 12, 829, 1984.
60. Polora, T., Bing, D., Mammel, M., and Boros, S., Neonatal high-frequency jet ventilation, *Pediatrics,* 72, 27, 1983.
61. Rock, J., Pfaelle, H., Smith, R. B., Mendelow, H., and Klain, M., High pressure jet insufflation used to prevent aspiration and its effect on the tracheal mucosal wall, *Crit. Care Med.,* 4, 135, 1976.
62. Jacobs, H. B., Emergency percutaneous transtracheal catheter and ventilator, *J. Trauma,* 12, 50, 1972.
63. Doyle, H. J., Napolitano, A. E., Lippman, R., Cooper, K. R., Duncan, J. S., Eakins, K., and Glauser, F. L., Different humidification systems for high-frequency jet ventilation, *Crit. Care Med.,* 12, 815, 1984.
64. McEvoy, R. D., Davies, N. J. H., Hedenstierna, G., Hartman, M. T., Spragg, R. G., and Wagner, P. D., Lung mucociliary transport during high-frequency ventilation, *Am. Rev. Respir. Dis.,* 126, 452, 1982.
65. Nordin, U., Keszler, H., and Klain, M., How does high frequency jet ventilation effect the mucociliary transport?, *Crit. Care Med.,* 9, 160, 1981.
66. Armengol, J. A., Man, S. F. P., Logus, J. W., Man, G. C., and King, E. G., Effects of high frequency oscillatory ventilation on canine tracheal mucous transport, *Crit. Care Med.,* 9, 192, 1981.

67. Ackerman, N. B., Jr., Null, D. M., Jr., and deLemos, R. A., High frequency ventilation: history, theory and practice, in *Respiratory Failure,* Kirby, R. R., Smith, R. A., and Desautels, D. A., Eds., Churchill Livingstone, London, 1985.
68. Faridy, E. E., Permutt, S., and Riley, R. L., Effect of ventilation on surface forces in excised dogs' lungs, *J. Appl. Physiol.,* 21, 1453, 1966.
69. Greenfield, L. J., Ebert, P. A., and Benson, D. W., Effect of positive pressure ventilation on surface tension properties of lung extracts, *Anesthesiology,* 25, 312, 1964.
70. Wyszogrodski, I., Kyei-Aboagye, K., Taeusch, H. W., Jr., and Avery, M. E., Surfactant inactivation by hyperventilation: conservation by end-expiratory pressure, *J. Appl. Physiol.,* 38, 461, 1975.
71. Williams, J. V., Tierney, D. F., and Parker, H. R., Surface forces in the lung, atelectasis, and transpulmonary pressure, *J. Appl. Physiol.,* 21, 819, 1966.
72. Massaro, G. D. and Massaor, D., Morphologic evidence that large inflations of the lung stimulate secretion of surfactant, *Am. Rev. Respir. Dis.,* 127, 235, 1983.
73. Faridy, E. E., Effect of distension on release of surfactant in excised dogs' lungs, *Respir. Physiol.,* 27, 99, 1976.
74. Hildegran, J. N., Goerke, J., and Clements, J. A., Surfactant release in excised rat lung is stimulated by air inflation, *J. Appl. Physiol.,* 51, 905, 1981.
75. Oyarzun, M. J. and Clements, J. A., Ventilatory and cholinergic control of pulmonary surfactant in the rabbit, *J. Appl. Physiol.,* 43, 39, 1977.
76. Nicholas, T. E. and Barr, H. A., The release of surfactant in rat lung by brief periods of hyperventilation, *Respir. Physiol.,* 52, 69, 1983.
77. Frantz, I. D., Stark, A. R., Davis, J. M., Davies, P., and Kitzmiller, T. J., High-frequency ventilation does not affect pulmonary surfactant, liquid or morphologic features in normal cats, *Am. Rev. Respir. Dis.,* 126, 909, 1982.
78. Mannino, F. L., McEvoy, R. D., and Hallman, M., Surfactant turnover in high frequency oscillatory ventilation, *Pediatr. Res.,* 16, 1661, 1982.
79. Ray, J. U., Goldberg, R. B., and Bland, R. D., Vibratory ventilation decreases filtration of fluid in the lung of newborn lambs, *Circ. Res.,* 52, 456, 1983.
80. Rehder, K., Schmid, E. R., and Knopp, T. J., Long-term high-frequency ventilation in dogs, *Am. Rev. Respir. Dis.,* 128, 476, 1983.
81. Todd, M. M., Toutant, S. M., and Shapiro, H. M., The effects of high-frequency positive-pressure ventilation on intracranial pressure and brain surface movement in cats, *Anesthesiology,* 54, 496, 1981.
82. Raju, T. N. K., Braverman, B., Nadkarny, U., Kim, W. D., and Vidyasagar, D., Intracranial pressure and cardiac output remain stable during high frequency oscillation, *Crit. Care Med.,* 11, 856, 1983.
83. Toutant, S. M., Todd, M. M., Drummond, J. C., and Shapiro, H. M., Cerebral blood flow during high frequency ventilation in cats, *Crit. Care Med.,* 11, 712, 1983.
84. Marquez, J., Guntupalli, K., Sladen, A., and Klain, M., Renal function and renin secretion during high frequency jet ventilation at varying levels of airway pressure, *Crit. Care Med.,* 11, 930, 1983.
85. Marquez, J. M., Douglas, M. E., Downs, J. B., Wu, W-H., Mantini, E. L., Kuck, E. J., and Calderwood, H. W., Renal function and cardiovascular responses during positive airway pressure, *Anesthesiology,* 50, 393, 1979.
86. Cornish, J. D., Coalson, J. J., Kuehl, T. J., and deLemos, R. A., Unpublished observations.
87. Bell, R. E., Coalson, J. J., Ackerman, N. B., Null, D. M., Kuehl, T. J., and deLemos, R. A., A nonpulmonary complication of high frequency oscillation, submitted for publication.
88. Busnell, L. S., Personal communication.
89. Bredenberg, C. E., Paskanik, A., and Fromm, D., Portal hemodynamics in dogs during mechanical ventilation with positive end-expiratory pressure, *Surgery,* 90, 817, 1981.
90. Mitzner, W., Effect of portal venous pressure on portal venous inflow and splanchnic resistant, *J. Appl. Physiol.,* 37, 706, 1974.
91. Moreno, A. H., Burchell, A. R., Van Der Woude, R., and Burke, J. H., Respiratory regulation of splanchnic and systemic venous return, *Am. J. Physiol.,* 213, 455, 1967.
92. Shiraki, K., Hepatic cell necrosis in the newborn. A pathologic study of 147 cases, with particular reference to congenital heart disease, *Am. J. Dis. Child.,* 119, 395, 1970.
93. Weinberg, A. G. and Bolande, R. P., The liver in congenital heart disease, *Am. J. Dis. Child.,* 119, 390, 1970.
94. Coen, R. and McAdams, A. J., Visceral manifestation of shock in congenital heart disease, *Am. J. Dis. Child.,* 119, 383, 1970.
95. deLemos, R. A. and Null, D. M., Personal observation.

INDEX

A

B

C

D

E

F

G

H

I

J

K

L

M

U

V

W

Z